Thank you

Ken K. McQueen

Hey Ross,

My foray into the creative process. Satisfying doesn't begin to describe it.

Dave Hutchinson

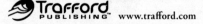

in memory of

Jocelyne Lois Hutchinson
June 14, 1933 – March 17, 2006

"winnie the gram" formally known as "the ticket" also known as "mum."

for

**my daughter, Emma Jane and
my wife, Shelly shelly bo belly**

acknowledgements

A major theme in this memoir is my passion
for the "Document." I would be remiss if I did
not acknowledge the role Arlene Keis and Bob
Earp had in my personal development in the
field of training.

I would also like to acknowledge the leadership
role of Gary McMillan. Your preparation
for Winnipeg's first marathon in 1979 has
provided me with a lifetime of inspiration.

epigram

A good plan, violently executed now, is better than a perfect plan next week.

George S. Patton

US general (1885 - 1945)

Contents

Introduction

It was day one of my running initiative. My hands were clammy and my tongue hurt like no tomorrow. The date was November 1, 2002, and I was in a deep double knee bend as I held my hands, palms down, fingers wide, over the glowing amplifier tubes of my stereo. I tested my dexterity by slightly shifting my weight forward onto my toes. My eyes remained fixed on the glass-encased red filaments, and my hovering hands were steady as they absorbed the radiating heat. I was waiting for a Diana Krall CD to load so that I could adjust the volume control to an optimum listening level before straightening out and reunifying my backside with the couch. Satisfied with the volume level, I rerouted my attention to fluffing a couple of oversize pillows and placing them strategically in one corner of the couch. Once I'd deposited myself into this sanctum and attained a proper lounging angle, I positioned the reading lamp, then placed a thick stack of newly printed eight and one half by eleven paper on my protruding belly. A red pen then appeared in my right hand from where, I don't know. Between my seven-year-old daughter and me, the house was littered with pens and pencils, much to my lovely wife's dismay.

An hour earlier I was having lunch in front of the computer screen, a three-cheese sandwich I guess four-cheese if you include the cheese bread. It was while I was munching away on this dairy concoction that I saw a series of grossly misspelled words. Shock of shocks, how could this be? Here I was, minutes away from printing and mailing off a reader's copy of my fiction manuscript, when the horrors of my carelessness caused me to lose control of my body functions and bite my tongue. A seldom-used vocalization process dealt with the searing pain in my mouth. While I randomly scrolled through the electronic pages, I determined that the problem was a combination of an overzealous spell-check function on the part of the word processor and complete ineptitude in its use on the part of yours truly. There were homonym problems and search-and-replace problems. I had asked the program to go to specific words and change them, but it had also changed a lot of other spellings of words that had the same pattern of letters in them.

I decided that it all came down to operator error, with the root cause being trying to perform a spell-check at two o'clock in the morning. Nodding off and clicking the "replace all" button is not recommended behaviour. So I reserved a large block of time to sit back, relax, and go through the printed manuscript manually, paper page by paper page. On the one hand this editing problem was unacceptable, while on the other hand it could be easily fixed with no creative writing involved and besides, it gave me an excuse to stretch out.

I picked the first of more than three hundred pages off my belly, but before I started scanning for errors, I held the page to the side so that I could admire my feet. Remember, this was day one of my running initiative. My brand-spanking-new runners were angled just off the couch at the ankle, and they were looking marvellous. I clapped them together a few times to add sound to the overall effect. I had purchased them that morning after seeing my wife off to work, walking my daughter to school, and then standing in line at the neighbourhood sporting goods store waiting for it to open. It wasn't as if they were having a door-crasher sale or an oversized inflatable gorilla bearing a clearance sign had lured me there. I was just eager. Price was no object as long as I didn't feel I had paid too much. So the lineup consisted of me and only me. Some days nothing feels better than being number one.

I last bought runners just a couple of years before my daughter Emma was born. If I wasn't starting up this whole running initiative and all, I probably would have made them last for ten years. Obviously, I don't embrace making change for change's sake, and I sure don't do a heck of a lot of physical activity.

I don't do a lot of shopping either, so when I trooped off to the sporting goods store I knew I would be susceptible to feature-laden, know-it-all salespeople and their finely honed, mind-controlling, high-pressured sales pitches. To counteract this inexperience, I took my standard evasive action of getting in and out with extreme promptitude. Although I did take the smallest of moments to stand in front of the great wall of right-foot-only footwear and absorb the power of athleticism that emanated from it. Or I could have been absorbing the heat of the high-intensity lighting and feeling the immense pressure of knowing that a salesman was probably closing in on my backside.

Whatever the case, I extended my fingers and filled my lungs with the scent of rubber and lace. I then spun on the outboard-sloped heel of my runner and picked up from a neatly stacked clearance pile what I thought would be the next and possibly last runners of this Hutchinson generation. I left without lacing them up or giving myself the opportunity to stand in front of a mirror and admonish myself for not getting what few hairs I had remaining cut last week. The success of my shopping experience was gauged by the fact that I had to hold the door open on my way out for the employees taking out the sidewalk racks now that's a man of action!

And my new runners sure clapped good. The sound was thick and solid, with the proper amount of decay in the acoustically dampened living room. Pings, echoes, and rattling picture frames were not permitted in this environment. The runners' genuine sound performance was enhanced by their drop-dead looks. The bright white, solid leather uppers and subtle off-white stitching with matching rubber soles dazzled me and left me lusting in anticipation of their first polishing.

After listening to them a few more times, my only complaint was that the laces seemed a bit thick and their plastic tips seemed a little long. I considered this to be a quality control issue. The extra length in the lace tips clicked and clacked as I clapped the runners together. I was a little worried about the annoyance factor when I put it in gear and was cruising down the street. In my mind the sound I created would be strong, powerful, and unrelenting, like the white noise of a machine working diligently in the background. I remember thinking that if these laces made me sound like a live-performance ad for the next Riverdance production, I would toast them, there was no doubt about it.

One hour easily slipped into another as I continued to scrutinize my homophones and clap my runners. These simple tasks allowed my mind to drift to mile upon mile of open road running. I was thinking really hard about running, and just as the fall-afternoon reading light degraded, I realized I was sweating. No, I hadn't broken into a cold sweat because I had to pick Emma up from school. Her friend's mother was picking up my littler one on that day. But if I had forgotten, it wouldn't have been the first time. No, the sweat was a hot and bothersome wetness, and much to my dismay it was coming from my feet.

The spell-checking came to a halt as I considered this turn of events. How could this be? I had done sweet nothing. I hadn't even tightened the laces for action at the highest levels of athletic achievement. Maybe more to the point, I hadn't really stood up in them yet. I then stared at my feet, full time. After considering such things as the room temperature, my craving to polish the leather, my coloured socks, and the time of day, I concluded that I had purchased a fine pair of outdoor café loungers. Together with a designer-branded cappuccino track suit, I could project a daring yet dashing image in Vancouver's West End on Denman Street. But I didn't own a track suit,

I didn't live in the West End, daring Dave was an oxymoron, and the last thing I needed was more lounge time.

After my hands were finished their airborne theatrics (with the accompanying gasps of "Why?"), I got them to unlace and box the runners. If I took pills, this would have been a good time to take one; instead, I hold frank conference calls with myself to myself about myself. I used to be quite self-conscious about talking out loud during these calls, but modern technology has provided relief in this area. The invention of the hands-free cellphone has semi-legitimized my involuntary manner of coping with stress. I now blend in with the masses well, at least those with arm movements from the Toller Cranston figure skating era. This blending in has the added benefit of deterring any accidental carting off in the paddy wagon.

My frank conference call continued in the car all the way back to the sporting goods store, and I didn't feel the need to look over my shoulder once. Yes, I would request a sales associate. Yes, I would listen to everything he or she told me. No, I would not argue with him or her. Yes, I would answer at least two questions about myself. Yes, I would try on more than one pair of shoes. Yes, I would accept the fact that I may have to wear a logo, possibly a known one. No, I would not debate with the sales associate while under the pretense of inquiring minds want to know. Oh, the horror, the horror of it all. I wished Shelly was at my side to guide me through the retail process with her firm yet reassuring shut-ups and not nows.

Once the car was parked, I put up the convertible roof and smiled at the anomalous November blue sky through a gaping hole in the fabric. I then momentarily let my thoughts meander as the roof approached my head on the way down. It landed with its usual loud and undignified slam against the top of the windshield, and a smattering of water hit my face from topside through the hole. My smile didn't completely diminish because I was amusing myself with thoughts of which bridge this pile of junk would break down on for some unsuspecting auto thief, who would have no problem slipping a hand through the hole, unlocking the door, and making off.

As I pulled out my glass-cleaning cloth and began to dry my eyeglasses, I grinned at the thought of renting my car to the Delta municipality as a bait car. My sales pitch would be the inexpensive anti-auto-theft angle. There would be no need to even wire the bait car for communication back to the police department when it was stolen. All they would need to do was listen to the local radio traffic updates for the breakdown of the black convertible on the Alex Fraser Bridge, again, then mobilize the force.

I grabbed the shoebox, slammed the heavy door closed, and was heading towards the sporting goods store when it crossed my mind that in the nearly twenty years I have had the car, it had never been stolen. This could be a problem. Isn't it a prerequisite of being a bait car that it be considered some sort of prize?

At this point I realized I had forgotten to lock the door, so I reversed course back to the pile of junk. I guess I could have left it unlocked, but what if it *did* get stolen? Shelly wouldn't be too happy with the bait car explanation. And how would she know? Well, Shelly has this auditor-like ability to find things out. I don't help matters any with my involuntary reflex action of giving everything up wholeheartedly in a vociferous spew whenever the auditor questions start flowing. This conditioned behaviour is from my former career in the aviation industry, where auditing in all its tentacled forms is a fact of life. Believe me, Shelly would think it entirely plausible that a successful bait car experiment took place. But that was not my real reason for locking the door. It had already been a bad week on the marital front because of a little VCR mix-up. I was locking the car door because losing our vehicle to a bait car experiment and not taping Shelly's favourite soap opera in the same week would put too much of a strain on the entire household, which includes the littlest member, the dog.

Since I broke my key off in the lock not last decade but the one before that, I need to lock the darn door by opening it and reaching far in towards the hinges and manually pushing the flimsy plastic knob lock. There are two reasons I abhor doing this. The first is I prefer not to bend over. If you are not thin and slim, then bending over just isn't one of your preferred activities. Shelly and Emma always hide Christmas presents, chocolate doughnuts, and Halloween candy on the lowest of shelves, of course with the accompanying conspiratorial whispers of "He'll never, ever look here." The second reason is that opening the closed door, sticking my head in the car interior, and breathing in the mildew and rotting canvas odour of the convertible top just isn't enticing. Let me tell you, at least in my case, driving with the top down is the preferred driving mode because you don't have to smell it.

Anyway, after depressing my chubby cheek on the top of the driver's side window because I was trying my hardest not to bend over or put my head in the car, I got the door locked. I then let my breath out, attempted to rub out the crease in my face, clutched the shoebox under my arm, and marched with supreme confidence towards the store. The spring in my step surprised me because on the rare occasions that I return merchandise, I normally drift in with my hands held high for utmost visibility. Usually I take the easy way out and just purchase a second item, really. I could go on about my personal return policy and its far-reaching benefits to mankind, but to sum it up quickly, I have this fear of being charged with shoplifting when I re-enter the store with said goods.

Once I got inside the store, a strapping young salesman made eye contact with me, and I didn't scurry away in the opposite direction or close my eyes and hope he was not there when I opened them. Instead, I held out the boxed runners in one hand and the receipt in the other as a sort of peace offering. He gave me a big toothy smile and, much to my relief, took the goods out of my hands. There would be no charges pending today—well, at least until I selected a new pair.

The salesman listened to my explanation of the leather material being inappropriate, then he nodded approvingly when I said I wanted him to personally work with me in selecting another pair of runners. Up to that moment, it had been so far so good as I capitulated my standard purchasing behaviour in order to move the running initiative ahead in a positive manner.

The salesman walked me over to the great wall of right-foot-only footwear but it didn't take long before my new-found euphoria began to wane as I realized I was not really part of the process here. I expected the athletic lad to get me involved by asking a few incisive questions, then engage in some back and forth banter in which he would slowly extol the benefits I would receive from his hand-selected runners. I also expected that by the time the closing pitch was made, I would have an urgent primordial need to put them on and run like the wind. You know, the mind control stuff. Instead, I got a loquacious technical information download that left my head lolling from shoulder to shoulder. He was a nice guy and all, but if I didn't have such a deep commitment to my running initiative, I would have walked. Instead, I felt a bit deflated and sat down while he droned on.

I'm not sure if the lights were making me sweat again or if it was residual water from the convertible roof, but as I was wiping whatever it was from my brow, the salesman caught my attention with a medical-sounding utterance. I had never been given the pitch of getting some sort of disease if I didn't buy a certain product. I began to formulate a series of questions about the symptoms he described as a spontaneous contraction of the muscles when I caught myself, took a deep breath, sat back, and relaxed. My question formulation process usually ends up in some sort of debate or at the very least in getting completely off subject. I took another deep breath and asked to try on the medical-miracle wonders instead of debating the veracity of the pitch. I could feel the air conditioning cooling the back half of my wide-open eyes when the salesman's reply included my first name.

INTRODUCTION

Maybe the lad had more sales savvy—no doubt through the in-store training system—than I had first thought.

My goodness they felt great. Right out of the box they were, easily the best-fitting shoes I'd ever tried on. I took a few small steps and found that the lightweight design made me feel as if I had lost a few pounds already. Remarkable! The price of the blue-toned beauties on the great wall caught my attention during this initial step test. I then calculated the benefits of the perceived weight loss and their purported ability to ward off disease and came to the conclusion that being double the cost of the pair I was returning was well worth it. The cashier close-out of the sale went smoothly, but it was a little unnerving having the manager, two cashiers, and the salesman all coming on as if they'd known me for years. My early-morning foray must have left more of an impression than I had intended it to. I exited the sporting goods store and scanned the flat expanse of the suburban parking lot, and once I determined that my car hadn't been stolen, I declared the first day of my running initiative an outstanding success.

The next morning under a ridge of high pressure, I walked in a stiff and forced manner on the way back from Emma's school. I knew that once I got back home the deed was going to be done. I was going to go running, and my body language indicated that the situation was grave. I knew this because as I visualized the rest of the morning, I took note that there were no Toller Cranston arm movements during this walk; I was more than just tense.

Rosie, our little Lhasa apso–poodle cross, greeted me at the door with a rare propeller tail wag. I paused only momentarily to give Rosie a scratch and accept a few licks because I didn't want to break the momentum of the morning's mission. I donned the blue-toned beauties, grey sweatpants, and a grey T-shirt and grabbed a glass of Delta's artesian-well blended tap water.

I began my warm-up based on archived memories that hadn't been accessed for absolute ages. The feeling of gloom and doom descended upon me again very early into the second set of exercises,

19

which ironically turned out to be a good thing since this lengthened my warm-up time. Sit-ups, push-ups, knee bends, leg lifts, hamstring stretches, groin stretches all the memories of Prime Minister Trudeau's era of guilt-ridden exercise regimens and the accompanying Liberal government propaganda were coming back strong and free as I worked out in the living room. At the end of the third set, my heart was pounding away in my chest as the image of some sixty-year-old Swede casually doing jumping jacks overtook my mind's eye. Thirty years later that Swede from the federal government indoctrination films, with his effortless form, was still getting my dander up.

I grabbed another glass of water and let the pounding in my chest ease up to a point where I could hear Rosie's nails clicking on the cork flooring in the kitchen. As I shook my head at the dog to indicate that she wasn't about to go for a walk, the feelings of dread were replaced with the contentment of having accomplished the first part of the plan. The rest of the plan included actually getting out the door and going for a short jaunt around the trail in the neighbourhood park, which is a part of the Sungod Recreation Centre. Just once around. I realized I was out of shape and that this was sort of like day one of training camp. The plan for after the morning session was to plan for the afternoon session. I figured I would take a conservative approach and soak in the tub for a few hours while I formulated the next session based on my morning performance.

I closed and locked the back door, then stood looking at my hand. The plan didn't include what to do with a fistful of keys and no pockets to put them in. But before this became a showstopper, my feet inexplicably began to move towards the back gate. By the time the back gate had closed, perpetual motion had taken me down the driveway, and my head had just figured out what my feet had already known: my hand would carry the keys.

Beyond the driveway lay the path to my running initiative. It would start off on the roadway since the side streets don't have sidewalks in this part of Delta. By the time my second foot had touched the roadway, I had looked left and right to see if anyone was watching, then by the third step I was off and running.

Thank goodness no one was out, especially any Swedish joggers. I figured I was two weeks of two-a-day workouts away from taking on the Swedes. Oh, back in the day I had met Prime Minister Trudeau's challenge. As a youngster I wore gold cleats and easily surpassed all those Swedish benchmarks that the phys. ed. teachers dutifully checked off on their clipboards. Still, I never did do any head-to-head competition with any old foreigners, and the image seemed a bit fearful at that moment so I checked around again. All was clear, but I wish I could say the same about my lungs. I was thirty feet away from the driveway, and I could probably still smell my car if I could only breathe. As I got to the second house down, my gasping had stopped, but only because I was now holding my breath. My arms and chest were starting to bulge as I muscled my way down the street.

Just around the nearest corner is the eighth house from my driveway. At this point in my run to the park, I looked down at the blue-toned beauties for answers to this unanticipated struggle, and then in the very next step I went from running to walking. The transition was instantaneous and life-saving. It brought release from such unusual and unnatural activities as clenching my teeth and not breathing. I figured I had averted asphyxia by milliseconds.

With my senses and faculties dulled, I stumbled forward, not knowing what was going to happen next since this wasn't part of the morning plan. I wasn't running, but again inexplicably my feet kept moving. My stupefaction had not lessened by the time I reached the intersection of 112th Street and 80th Avenue. The red traffic light allowed me to stop, remove my glasses, rub my eyes, and bend over. My hand then spasmed open as my wrist met my knee at an awkward angle, and the keys jangled as they hit the cement. As I bent over further to pick them up, the car making a tight right turn in front of me almost shattered my eardrums as it screeched to a sudden stop. I suppose he thought I was about to dive under his wheels. Yeah, whatever. I then felt the stares of all the motorists who were at the intersection, their faces radiating pity.

Now with relatively all my senses in failure mode, I drew my back up straight and began the resuscitation process by putting my glasses back on. With the cars stopped, turned heads and all, I heard through the cacophony of profanity and the sounds of the great outdoors one single line: "Throw in the towel, buddy, you're gonna hurt yourself."

Wishing to escape this focal point of attention, I faced the blue sky, wiped the sweat from my brow, and watched the stark red traffic light suspended by a single slight cable gently waiver in the breeze. I didn't dare look down and take responsibility for the scene; instead I found it easier and much less humiliating to turn and walk in the direction of home. I had run a quarter of a kilometre and maybe staggered another quarter and that was it. The simple, plangent fact being that I was spent.

The walk down the block on the way back home was as much of a mental struggle as the run had been physically. I glanced furtively into each living room window, attempting to identify all possible witnesses to such an inglorious conclusion to my jaunt through the park. I was able to shake this initial embarrassment when the cooling of my sweat resulted in a wicked case of the shivers, which had me in survival mode by the time I opened the back door at home.

Once inside there was no fanfare from Rosie. The little dog had obviously curled up and gone to sleep somewhere, not expecting me back so soon. To top it off, I didn't feel like a returning conquering hero as I scampered to the bathroom and fought a losing battle with the shower curtain when I misjudged the opening in my desperate attempt to get the hot water running. Minutes later I lay in the tub with the mirror reassuringly steamed over, even where the curtain and rod were propped haphazardly against it. Those new spring-loaded rods just don't stand up to the rigours of a man trying to better himself.

Once the heat of the water stopped the shivering, I put my reinvention of the curtain rod on hold and began the analysis of what in the world could have caused such shame and humiliation this morning. My plan looked good from the point of view that I had figured the living would be easy and I would be in the tub at this point. I just hadn't imagined that being in the tub would be out of dire necessity. Also if the highlight of the plan was taking a bath well, that was pretty weak.

Most other aspects of the morning run were weak as well. The inability to even get a glimpse of the park let alone run though it, the burning lung issue, the clothing situation, the lack of pockets, and the whole fear of exposing my vulnerabilities to the living rooms of the neighbourhood. The absurd notion of someone even thinking I was attempting suicide was weak. Now there was a person who gets my nomination for a full round of therapy. As I towelled off I remembered that my left heel felt uncomfortable in the blue-toned beauties, and considering that they were my second pair of runners, that was weak as well.

After rummaging through an unruly pile of monotone fabrics on a chair in the bedroom, I slipped into some dry and customarily oversized clothing. I then retreated to the living room to continue my analysis. There were some positives, the first being the warm-up session. There was good variation in the exercises over a reasonably long duration of time. Getting my heart rate up during the warm-up and then cooling down just before the run I checked off as real positives as well.

The biggest and most surprising positive was my attitude. The ease with which I got myself out the door surprised me, something I contributed to a healthy state of mind towards day two of the running initiative. But the bouquet side of the ledger was short, and it didn't take long before I was entrenched in the beef side of the ledger. The overwhelming evidence of my complete lack of physical conditioning was astonishing. Oh, I knew I had been out of the sweat and grunt mode of fitness for a while—it could probably be measured in years if I cared to add it up—but the profundity of the infinitesimal level I seemed to be at was crushing.

A sense of anger overcame me as I reviewed each laborious step from the morning's failed attempt, which drove me to the kitchen to soothe myself with a hot lunch. It was during lunch that I began a review of the footwear and the uncomfortable sensation I had felt in my left heel. I donned the blue beauties again, this time with suspicion, and gave them a few test flexes while I ate. Sure enough, there was a problem with the left shoe. Every time I put pressure on the left heel it felt uncomfortable, as if the stitching was bad or some other form of poor product quality. I tested the foot out of the shoe on the cork floor, and it felt fine. It was definitely the shoes. The blue beauties had seduced me with their elegant lines, soft interior contours, and wonderful rich colour, but they were defective. Well, that explained a lot.

I didn't even finish eating, and the chair lurched when I gave it an indignant push away from the table. I grabbed the offending sportswear, wet-wiped their bottoms, and chucked them into their box before heading back to the sporting goods store. Maybe for the first time in my life I had no trepidation as I strode into the retail store, flagging down a young salesperson using my best Toller Cranston arm movements. I then placed the source of all my problems on the counter and instructed the young woman that the selection process was about to begin yet again.

Moments later as I stood before the great wall of right shoes, I heard an older woman's voice directly over my shoulder. She was so close that her breath was intrusive, like an active sonar ping from a battleship. With little room to manoeuvre, I was forced to pivot on the balls of both feet. As the older woman informed me that she was the store manager, the younger saleswoman retreated a few steps to the relative safety of a metal display case that was taller than she was. The virago with the boxed blue-toned beauties tucked up under her fleshy arm then demanded to know my biggest problem with the product. I didn't hesitate as I told her how the inferior runners she held had ruined my day. The rebuttal centred on getting me out of the store with the exact same shoes; after all, this was my second merchandise return and she was not amused.

Pretty much on any other day of my time spent alive she would have been successful in stemming my retail insurgence, but not on this day. I was adamant that a glue line, shoddy stitching, or a void in the moulded rubber sole was a problem and that as a result I had suffered great anguish. She was lucky I didn't sue for loss of a morning's pleasure. After much jostling of the shoe between us, complete with multiple finger probes of its interior, I may have been caving somewhat when I pointed to a more expensive model on the great wall of shoes as an example of superior fit and finish. This seemed to placate the pugnacious manager, and she quickly beckoned the younger salesperson over with her preferred probing finger. As the manager retreated to some overlord position beyond my vision, the salesperson directed me to sit down and chill out. Then she asked, "Do you really run?"

I sat there humped over and all hot and bothered from my conversation with the manager. I could feel my gut pinching on my belt buckle and an upper body strain between my shoulder blades, no doubt caused by jostling the shoe back and forth. I meekly sighed an "Oh, yeah" as I slipped off my shoes in anticipation of starting the dreaded fitting process.

The young salesperson laughed and said, "Are you sure?" before walking away to get my size from who knows where, because it looked as if she was heading to the ladies section. What type of retail lunacy had I gotten myself into? I swear I would have eaten the costs up to this point and walked right there and then if I had been wearing my shoes and if I hadn't been so exhausted from the morning's physical endeavour.

Anyway, the young woman came back, and I tried on the runners that I had just blindly pointed to during the heat of the argument. Wow, they felt totally cool. I was told they had more panels for ventilation than any other shoe on the wall. The coolness equated to lightness as I walked around a bit then headed towards the cashier, leaving my old runners under the fitting bench. The salesperson scrambled to catch up with me and asked if she could box the shoes, just as the manager showed up with a cashier. I pulled out my credit card and told her I wouldn't need a box this time around. In my mind I knew I'd never be able to handle the stress of returning these cool runners. Besides at these prices, if they didn't work out, what would?

Once my feet felt the cool November outdoor air I knew instantly that I was wearing a shoe with a purposeful design. All in all I wouldn't say these mesh-panelled babies had a lot of flash, but I felt confident that this time I had gotten some dash—even if they cost me more than three times the price of my original purchase.

The next morning I woke up with thoughts of effortlessly running to the park in my new runners. Then with a grunt and a roll that took maximum effort, I managed to get my roly-poly body to the edge of the bed. With my usual bounce, always much to Shelly's dismay, I was out of bed and ready for action.

In my first step of the day I encountered blazing pain in my left foot that left me groaning and grasping the polished armoire for upright support. My left heel felt as if it had been shattered or at the very least beaten and bruised. My great mass thumped over to the light switch on one foot with such earthquake force that loose items such as jewellery jangled and entertainment controls vibrated. I flipped the switch, Shelly bolted upright in bed, and her query of whether I had stepped on our little dog was just this side of hysterical. I didn't answer; I was too busy in my struggle to lift my foot up to the light in an attempt to gain visual confirmation of what surely had to be horrific to look at.

In hopping around I had transversed the room a second time, and as my ample butt banged against the armoire in my desperate exploration for support, the armoire's looped metal latches clanged hard in confirmation. Finally, with the steadying influence of a solid mahogany joint at my back, I was able to get my first good look at the cause of such extraordinary pain.

I could hear Shelly alternating between soothing, whispering words to the dog and sharp-pointed questions directed my way since I really hadn't identified what the whole commotion was all about. And truthfully, after staring at the appendage in question and giving it a few managerial pokes with my finger, I still couldn't satisfy my wife's crack-of-dawn queries. First off, there was no blood either gushing out or pooling under the wrinkled white surface of the skin. There was no swelling, and incredibly there were no signs of protruding bones or embedded foreign objects. Although I hadn't ruled out the onslaught of some rare disease that certainly would take my life, I figured I owed Shelly the most logical explanation up to that very moment. "I think I've hurt myself running."

"*Running?* I've known you for more than ten years. You don't run," said Shelly. This was followed by a few strokes of the little dog's head and then a skeptical, "No way."

Obviously I hadn't gotten around to telling her about my whole running initiative, and I didn't feel like getting into it at that moment, so I limped off down the stairs to the living room couch.

The comfort of the couch and the solitude of the early morning afforded me the proper frame of mind to further assess my running injury and the whole initiative itself. Yes, I was quite confident that yesterday's morning run was the source of my pain. I didn't know the exact nature of the problem, but the more I thought about it, the clearer one part of the equation became. The shoes weren't the problem, any of them. This fact was mulled over until it consumed all my thoughts. With a review of each excursion to the sporting goods store, my embarrassment grew greater and greater.

The embarrassment eventually levelled off at my last great retail fiasco an incident at a big-box hardware store that resulted in the store's evacuation because of the smoke from a fire that, well, was linked to me. The fire, which occurred outside the store, was an accident, a little exothermic reaction that got out of hand, really. Shelly feared that if I ever ventured under the hardware store's big welcome sign again, I would never come out. As if they had my picture up on a most-wanted wall or something and I would be placed immediately into custody under a dizzying display of red flashing lights, complete with a disembodied voice warning of my threat status to all who bothered to listen. Because of this she was emphatic that I never step foot in that retail outlet again. I was just coming off a one-year boycott of the entire North American chain, so fulfilling her request for one store would be easy. To the best of my knowledge, the boycott, which is another story and the fire are not related.

Anyway, like the hardware store, I wouldn't be going back to the big-box sporting goods store. I just couldn't stand to look any of them in the eye. I thought at the time that they must think I'm simply out of my mind, bonkers style. I must admit I probably thought so too because later that morning over coffee I told Shelly everything. This included the name of the sporting goods store and the directive that if it should burn down in the next little while she should make contact with someone, exactly whom I didn't know. The scary part was how she took the news without even lifting her head from its oblique viewing position of her steaming coffee cup and how readily she agreed. It was as if she'd had the number secreted away in her purse for years.

It was while I sat on the couch giving my heel a gentle rub that another warning sign became evident. The partially opened shutters let in a soft blanket of morning light, revealing my new runners sitting askew in a corner by the left speaker. The left runner was on its side, and the right runner sat pigeon-toed towards it. This just wasn't right. I never leave my shoes in a pile or tossed about. They may not be in the closet as Shelly would like them, but they are always lined up neatly side by side wherever they end up. The illumination of the untested runners grew with intensity as the sun aligned with the shutters moment by moment to create a crisp white spotlight upon them. Although the clarity of the light and the positioning of the mesh-panelled babies afforded me the opportunity to admire their intrinsic details, all I could think of was Poh-Poh.

Poh-Poh was well known locally as an elderly Chinese grandmother who, as the fictional story goes, lived with her son and his young family in Vancouver's downtown east side during the Depression years of the 1930s. Poh-Poh was born in the southern Canton region of China, and when she immigrated to Canada she brought with her the culture and customs of China's house-servant women. This included having rituals and superstitions as an important part of her daily life. Poh-Poh believed that ghosts and spirits live among us and shape our destinies. I am certain that Poh-Poh would have seen the shoes in a heap in the corner as an ominous sign of bad fortune. That morning, the longer I sat there staring into the corner, the more I had to agree with Poh-Poh. I saw the shoes as the carnage from a train wreck, completely off the rails, going nowhere fast and as it turned out, neither was I. I didn't run again for two months.

The Document

After reading the Arts and Life section of the *Vancouver Sun* newspaper, I folded it in on itself then drew my arm up in a windmill fashion and slammed the paper down on the antique kitchen table well, really old, loosely assembled harvest table. Its leaves shook violently while its legs compressed under the initial impact, then sprung back with such force that the entire wooden structure became airborne. The flight didn't break anything, not even last summer's height or distance records that I set while squashing a mosquito. Maybe the flight was all of a thirtieth of an inch in height and a sixteenth of an inch in distance, but it was enough to frighten the little dog that just happened to be under the table into a wheezing and coughing fit. Rosie does this when she either gets too excited or, as in this case, too scared. While waiting for the worst of the coughing to subside, I sat at the table and unfolded the newspaper to the article I had been reading. I then picked up the little dog and apologized profusely as I prepared to reread the piece.

The article in the *Vancouver Sun* was about running. Specifically, it was about training to run the Vancouver Sun Run, which the newspaper has sponsored since 1985. I'd never run the Sun Run, of course, but back in its early days I used to live one block off of the run route in Vancouver's West End. It never ceased to amaze me at how peaceful my sleep could be while a mass of early-morning physical fitness maniacs surged along the shore of English Bay in a display truly emblematic of Vancouver. I knew of this only from watching the evening news, and every year I was always inspired to promise myself I would get up early next year and watch the event. Full emphasis on *watch*. Anyway, it didn't matter because the thought was as fleeting as the Sun Run maniacs were swift on their feet, and I never, ever, even in a month of Sundays, participated as a spectator.

The bottom line was that back in those days it might have been easier to stay up later than it would have been to get up early, and I'm sure the same could be said for Shelly. I did not meet, speak to, or even lust after Shelly until 1992, but amazingly my blue-eyed sweetheart lived two apartment buildings down on the same street from me. My dad and two different sets of friends also lived on Harwood Street. For the uninitiated, Vancouver's West End is an eclectic urban high-density downtown neighbourhood with multi-residential high-rise apartment buildings, and of course it has more than one leafy green, tree canopied street. During quiet moments I often think back to those years in the hood, so to speak, and scan for any memory of my future wife who lived within bellowing distance. There isn't any so far, but I'm not a guy who gives up easily, especially when it intrigues me to no end just thinking about it.

Over the years I've remembered many faces from the old neighbourhood, and to my surprise I've seen many of these people walking around malls, sitting at bus stops, or eating in restaurants right here in the suburban community area of North Delta. No, I don't think they are following me, but I have contemplated booking time with a sociologist to discuss this specific development in population redistribution. Then again, I've also thought about the cost of this endeavour and the possible embarrassing consequences, such as being referred to a psychologist. Whether it's because of the former or the latter, I've since decided that I will get my advice regarding this question dispensed from a realtors kiosk at the mall. Although it's now taken years to assess and select the best realtors kiosk to assail,

I don't need to spend a fraction of that time figuring out what Shelly did during those same Sun Run years. Shelly slept in too.

Once Rosie had stopped coughing and the quivering was down to the odd spasm, I let her down on the floor. I then completed the groundwork for intense scrutiny of the editorial variety when I anchored the Document to the wooden table with both elbows. That's right, the Document. That day's *Vancouver Sun* contained much more than just mere articles. It contained supporting evidence of a claim. It contained proof in the form of a chart. It even spoke to me in a direct manner. Within the Document it said, "See you at the finish line." Once I combined that cheerful and optimistic last line with the mind-and-body unshackling first line of "Run 30 seconds," that's where I lost it and nearly killed the dog. I was now studying the fine print in between two of the most stirring sentences I'd ever read, and to use the Sun Run Document's stylistic, straightforward approach and plaintive text, I just had to say, "Wow."

"Run 30 seconds" was amusing, even titillating, but as I read further I found that the Document had a professional structure to it as well. I could feel the ebb and flow from the easy to difficult portions of the workouts. The tasks progressed from simplest to hardest. The workouts were detailed down to the very second of each workout day, complete with weekly and monthly requirements. This Document wasn't fooling around; it was powerful and had incredible focus. I could feel the time, effort, and expertise that oozed from it as I assessed its learning cycle. It had processes, which were used at the beginning of each workout, then repeated each time with incremental changes, not only completing the learning cycles but also building upon them at the same time. The text, in the form of a two-column chart with a written preamble and training tips at the end, was laid out in an easy-to-read fashion and even had some snap in the form of three colours and a graphic splash.

The heart of the plan was broken down into three-a-week workouts over the course of thirteen weeks that after the third reading still left me flabbergasted. I mean, for the twenty-fifth workout, why would you run for sixty-three minutes? Why not a rounded-off sixty? Why not a casual jog of about an hour? Why not for the twenty-fifth session just get out there and give it everything you've got? I mean really, what's with sixty-three minutes?

I found the minutia of this timing thing so intriguing that I wanted to go out that very day and run sixty-three minutes, then study the effects, which of course would have defeated the purpose of this well-designed Document. Besides, based on my last running experience, if I ran sixty-three minutes Shelly would be called down to the morgue. Her curled eyelashes would be pressed tight, her head dramatically looking up and away, setting free and extenuating her long, freshly flat-ironed blonde hair, and held in her hands with the button-red polished nails would be the little dog. The dog would then be thrust forward to study the effects of physical exertion and body identification. I suppose a fit of coughing from the quivering rat-faced mongrel would signal a positive identification.

I sure liked that day's Arts and Life section of the *Vancouver Sun* because it contained something I did not have. A plan. I thought I had a perfectly good running plan when I attempted my run to the park and back. I knew I needed good equipment, so I bought some shoes. I knew I shouldn't go too far the first time, so I planned a short outing to the park. I knew I would need to build up to athlete status, so I planned two-a-day workouts just like the B.C. Lions do in their football training camps. I knew all this, and after reading that day's *Vancouver Sun*, I also knew I really didn't have a plan, just the outline of one. It also hit home that the two months I spent recovering from my heel injury after my first attempt at running were directly attributable to my lack of proper planning.

What the Sun Run plan had that I didn't, at least for starters, was definition. It defined a process that had the goal of running ten kilometres as its conclusion. The definition of the process included outlining a sequence of activities and what happened in each and every one of them. Good stuff; no making it up as you go along.

The Sun Run plan was also measurable. It had end-of-process measures for each activity, including time and distance. This enabled you to see whether you were sticking to the plan or not. An added bonus of the Sun Run plan, something truly exceptional, was the inclusion of due dates. It wasn't just a thirteen-week schedule that you fit in wherever and whenever. It took this ambiguity out of the equation and put in due dates. For instance, week four started February 11, 2003. A lump formed in my throat at this attention to detail. This Sun Run stuff was shaping up to be some serious bit of business.

The plan also appeared to be stable. What I mean is that it seemed doable, whereas my original plan was all in my head and aspired to push the boundaries of human endeavour after the first day. The Sun Run plan was completely documented and just seemed logical in format. It had conservative daily objectives, which gave me the feeling that I would be able to accomplish them. There is no better feeling than reading and instantaneously feeling good about whatever you just read.

As good as the Sun Run plan was, it did lack a few components. A feedback cycle was one of them, so I got up from the kitchen table, grabbed a pair of scissors from the kitchen drawer, and cut the Document out of the newspaper. I then dipped into Emma's arts basket for some glue, and I pasted the Document to a blank sheet of eight and a half by fourteen paper. Then it was back to Emma's basket for a ruler, which I used to draw a line beside each of the daily workout steps. This provided a commentary section, which I could later use to hold a team meeting, hopefully without conflict between my body and my mind, in an attempt to improve my performance. I wish I could take credit for this last part of the plan, but no, once again the Document did everything. So even if it didn't have a built-in feedback cycle, it told you to create one, at least in my interpretation it did. The last line in the training tips section said to keep a log.

Now who in the world would fall in love with a technical document? An overweight, balding, bespectacled office guy in his mid-forties who just got laid off from his human resource job in the aviation industry, that's who. The aviation industry's baseline is technical documents. In the pre-computer era, it was said that an aircraft didn't fly until it had an equivalent weight in paperwork. The purpose of the paperwork was to substantiate the manufacturing and regulatory processes. I suppose this nugget of wisdom would incorporate computer hard drives in today's manufacturing world, but I don't think the expression has ever been updated. Whatever the case, I'd spent twenty-five years of my adult life reading, writing, sourcing, and using technical and business documents. The breadth of my document experience includes but is not limited to aircraft drawings, ISO standards, quality control policies, collective bargaining agreements, company policy, and manufacturing standards from all of the major North American aviation manufacturers.

The question of who would love a document is easy to answer. The question of why that person would fall head over heels for a document about running, with complete capitulation to its methods, objectives, and outcomes, is much harder to answer. Obviously my health had come under scrutiny and I had decided to do something about it, but I honestly don't know why. Over the years my problem-solving skills have taught me that it is rare if not impossible for there to be one single answer for why a manufacturing process failed. So it's difficult to pin down why the poorly dressed, out of shape guy came running out of his house.

Certainly not the root cause but a good start to answering that question goes back to Poh-Poh. Poh-Poh is the fictional grandmother character in Wayson Choy's novel *The Jade Peony*, which won the 1996 City of Vancouver Book Award. There is no doubt in my mind that Poh-Poh, who spent her last years in Vancouver's Chinatown watching for signs of her death, would have interpreted the phone calls I received after I got laid off with their common theme of watch your health as a sign. A sign so bad that maybe it would be a good idea to never answer the phone again, and to be doubly sure that fate was not tempted, I should throw out the answering machine too. Well, Grandma, maybe back in old China you could do without a phone, but not in this country. "Old way, best way" not better this time.

So, based on the phone calls I received after I got laid off, it had become evident that my mum and sister, my peers, and a few ex-bosses all seemed to have taken the same truth serum and were concerned about my health. Hey, I wasn't. It was the last thing on my mind, although my doctor once told me I looked like a gorilla, which moved the weight issue up a notch in my mind but very temporarily since the rubber glove made an immediate and snappy appearance after the comment. I'd never had high cholesterol, my blood pressure had never been high, and my back was feeling the best it had in years. I'd never been hospitalized, even during the seventies when I had boogie fever. I was very content with my health, although I must admit I didn't stand too long in front of a mirror anymore.

I tried to shake off the comments of "Watch your health" as just an expression. You know, like "Good luck, pal" or something along those lines, where the words are tossed about in a casual and effortless manner with little thought. I tried, but thoughts of what the fatalistic Poh-Poh would say wouldn't let me. The sinking feeling that maybe the phone calls were a harbinger of an imminent health crash had taken over, and maybe just maybe I should deal with the reality side of life's ledger just a bit more. Anyway, that was my start to trying to answer the question of why I was so taken with the Document.

I got up from the table and rubbed my elbows to get rid of the flat spots in them. The start date for the Sun Run training program was that week, and now was as good a time as any to get the mesh-panelled babies back on. I hadn't worn them for a while because for some strange reason my left heel seemed to swell up just wearing them untied around the house. Fearing that I was developing a pain-by-association relationship with my runners, I ushered them to the back regions of the hall closet, where they joined other association outcasts from years gone by, such as some nearly new in-line skates. But that was in the past, and now after a very enjoyable two months off without any strenuous activity, my heel felt normal. This plus the official proclamation of my enrolment in the Sun Run training program—the Document was now attached to the fridge by magnets—meant that the mesh-panelled babies needed to be hauled out and laced up.

Later that evening, Shelly, Emma, and I, with our shoulders hunched and our fleece-lined jackets pulled high up around our necks, stepped silently through the winter drizzle on the way out to my car. When I stole a glance in their direction as I was opening my door, I saw that they were both standing motionless some twenty feet back.

"No heat, no heat," cried a little figure and a littler figure, whose expressions were lost in the dismal light. That's right, I had forgotten that when it came to my car, they were good-weather passengers only; we would need to take Shelly's SUV for our trip into Vancouver. Our friends Hitoshi and Mitsou had invited us for dinner, and for us, this was one of the social events of the year. Hitoshi is a cook of the highest order. When an invitation comes, you don't ask in a crass manner what's being served and then make your decision, you humbly accept then spend the days ahead drifting in a dream state as you anticipate the exotic and exquisite tastes coming soon to a mouth near you.

Hours after another marvellous meal, Hitoshi and I were relaxing on the overstuffed leather sofa talking about, shock of all shocks, running. For some reason I thought I would be the one holding court, going on and on about running, but on this night it was Hitoshi. I was hanging on every word he said as he went into detail about some tag-team run in the Fraser Valley. Hitoshi was a definite maniac. After the Fraser Valley relay run we talked about his training regime, then he switched the topic to my shoes. Tonight was the mesh-panelled babies' outside debut. Oh, I could feel winter's wet chill through them, but I found this extremely gratifying because it reinforced the feeling I had about their tremendous heat dissipation properties.

To the best of my knowledge, Hitoshi had seen my runners for only a fraction of a second as I doffed them at the front door, but he knew everything about them. When he mentioned the picture on them, I had to stop him and ask, "What picture?" I wasn't about to parade around with someone's picture on my feet. I leaped from the couch, ran to the front door, and grabbed a shoe for closer inspection. Sure enough, inside the shoe on the heel of the sole insert was a picture of what looked like then Vancouver mayor Larry Campbell wearing his fedora. The longer I stayed there, holding the picture of my left sole to the meagre glow provided by a mist-shrouded street light that filtered through the door's bevelled lead-glass window, the more I realized that maybe I was mistaken. It could have been councillor Jim Green.

Sadly, our fun night out had to come to an end, and I drove the quiet and barren route home to North Delta, accompanied by the less-than-quiet snoring of my family. Emma, as usual, fell asleep before I had the transmission in drive, and Shelly nodded her head a few minutes longer, alternating between casting hard looks at my shoes and slowly closing her big blue eyes until she too softly fell asleep. This gave me some quality time to reflect on the evening.

The dinner had been, well, fine dining as usual, but the best part of the night had been talking to Hitoshi about running. I was pumped. I was ready for action. I was one highly motivated dude. Although Hitoshi was a maniac and there was no way I could run with him in the near future, he had sure been an inspiration today. The more I thought about the effects Hitoshi had on me, the more I came to realize what the Sun Run Document was missing. It didn't have my personal goals, which would then lead to the ability to motivate myself. After all, I couldn't rely on gourmet dinners and inspirational talks from Hitoshi for the next thirteen weeks.

I went to bed that night thinking once again about my motivation. I woke up the next morning still thinking about my motivation. This cycle continued for the entire day while I paced around the house, breaking in the mesh-panelled babies. My goal couldn't be weight loss could it? That was what the phone calls were really about, weren't they? If that was what my family and friends were really saying, then their goal couldn't be my goal. It just doesn't work that way. If your goal is someone else's idea of what is good for you, then you will never be able to motivate yourself to the fullest extent possible. You need to do it for yourself, not for someone else. Call it the experience of an older guy, but I've watched people dig deeper, fight harder, and stick with it longer if the idea is theirs. I used this same reasoning for not using the Sun Run de facto goal of "InTraining to run 10K." That would be their goal for me. A self-gratifying one, for sure, but it was not mine.

I paced some more, then did some light exercise while I reviewed other possible goals. Competition with the Jones's is always a good one. My first attempt at running gave me a taste of what was to come, and I have to tell you to count me out. At this point I was confident I would get running again, but I didn't feel or see any of the athleticism of old. There was a reason the golden cleats of my past were lost in the outside storage shed. Years of inactivity and a suspect back had dimmed the spark for physical competition. If someone else was bigger, faster, or stronger than I was, good for him.

Setting an example by being a good role model got more pace time than I expected it to. I worked it from a few different angles. My argument of not having someone else's goal or doing it for someone else didn't win out so easily this time. I guess because I have a young daughter, and being able to run around the block would be setting a good example for her. In the end, again because I'd had a taste of what was to come, I figured there were many other less strenuous and much safer ways to be a good role model.

General well-being or quality of life as a goal made it all the way through breakfast and lunch. I ended up dropping them because they weren't specific enough. Then I dropped getting more fresh air for the opposite reason it was too specific and limiting.

I worked through training for Terry Fox, my personal hero,

in short time as well. Terry asked only for participation, he hadn't insisted on people running; they could walk, cycle, roll, or skate. Once I decided that training to run for Terry wasn't the fit I was looking for, I got up and circled the second Sunday after the Labour Day weekend on the calendar. Not making training to run for Terry my high-level goal wouldn't stop my participation in the annual Terry Fox run.

Then the challenge of meeting a new and different goal came and went pretty fast. At this stage in my life, this particular method of motivation had worn its welcome mat threadbare. It wasn't long before I was stuck on weight loss again. In fact, the weight loss issue had been coming up about once every two hours. It just wouldn't go away, no matter how many times I dowsed it with the strongest of denials. The more I thought about weight loss, the more I thought of Marlon Brando in the movie *Apocalypse Now.*

I saw myself playing the part of the fat actor after eating, oh, probably the first calorie-restricted lunch. I would be lying down just as he was at the end, except I would be right there on the kitchen floor next to the fridge, weak from hunger and moaning Brando's lines: "The horror, the horror . . ." I just couldn't do the weight loss thing. I didn't have the will, the fortitude, or the courage to face such anguish.

In a moment of despair, I quit the Sun Run program. I just wasn't going to go down that road of discovery if the reason for running was losing weight. Not a chance. I quit, then turned off the music. The music always dies when all is not right. After quitting, I felt a strange sense of accomplishment. I mean, after all, I hadn't done anything for most of the day except think about my goal for running. At least quitting was a verifiable act.

Yes, the quitting part was easy, and standing at the living room window with my arms folded across my chest, watching raindrops being blown across the glass into huge spider webs by January's gusts, was even easier. Of course, it didn't take long before I was thinking about the Sun Run program again. As I stood there looking out through the ever-changing liquid webs, all the pieces for my running goal came together. Very nicely I must add.

It was as if quitting the Sun Run had injected an urgency into resolving my dilemma instead of doing away with it. The problem with the weight loss goal was twofold. Apart from being someone else's goal, it was just too darn big. It deserved to be dealt with by itself. Because of this I was reluctant to give it equal billing with another goal.

I knew from a high-level perspective that I wasn't going to muddy the process by setting multiple goals. I didn't want to give myself the opening to squeak out a win in the final analysis by picking and choosing positive aspects from multiple goals and calling the process successful. No, I was going to keep it as simple as possible. I would either run the Sun Run or I wouldn't. There would be no self-congratulating for completing three quarters of the training, losing a few pounds, and feeling good about the new state of my overall health. No, none of that. I was planning on winning from the very beginning; it would be all or nothing. The final judgment would be simple and harsh—I either succeeded or failed.

And what goal didn't I want weight loss to share the spotlight with? Fitness, to be honest. Long before the layoffs and the phone calls, I had been developing a craving for a physical test. I had been inactive for such a lengthy period that the urge from my near-dormant muscles and tendons seemed deep and primal. It was as if they were nearing a point of no return and were sending out one last desperate DNA-encoded SOS message. It is a testament to how pervasive and powerful the weight loss issue was that it could suppress my true needs and desires. I had known for a while that I needed to get out there, but unfortunately all my athletic training had been in team sports, which held no interest for me at this time in my life. This was another reason the Sun Run Document grabbed my attention that day: it had the option of being an individual sport.

I turned my back to the window, put on a Sarah McLaughlin

CD, fast-tracked to the song "Fear," and jacked up the volume. I then found my arms doing their best Toller Cranston moves as I walked to the kitchen and in one deft arm movement whisked the Sun Run Document off the fridge. Yes, weight loss would be another war, probably a hallucinogenic jungle war based on the early skirmishes. If that night's dream started with the opening credits of Shelly starring as Martin Sheen in *Apocalypse Now*, then I promised myself I would reconsider not only my running goal but also my entire life. Anyway, while the overcast sky was still illuminated, it was the personal glory of physical achievement that was stoking my running aspirations, and unlike my first attempt where I physically gave everything, this time would be different. I was going to give it my all.

I settled in at the kitchen table and adjusted the shutters for optimum light on the Sun Run Document. With a red pen, I spelled the word *fitness* just above the coloured graphic splash, then circled it. Underneath this goal I started the mission statement, once again in red ink. "I am going to attain a higher . . ." Who am I kidding? A higher what? Level of fitness? With the implication being that I already had some fitness? Yeah, right. I crossed out "a higher," which was half on the blank white paper and half on the clipped then centred and pasted Sun Run Document. I continued with "fitness by completing the Sun Run program, which includes the Sun Run 2003."

Using a black pen, I drew an arrow away from the word *fitness* and identified it as my goal. I then drew an arrow away from the word *program* and identified it as the plan. I drew a third arrow away from the words *Sun Run 2003* and identified this as the timeline. I held up the single piece of paper, which now contained a goal, mission statement, plan, timeline, training tips, and the feedback sections I had previously drawn in. With a sense of accomplishment, I attached it to the fridge.

All that was fine, but unfortunately, as much as I loved this Document it was still missing something. It lacked a strategy on how in the world I was going to actually do this. I grabbed another blank piece of paper and began writing in bullet-point form my implementation strategies. I had just completed my thirtieth when Shelly walked in the door. Shelly's holiday season stretched into the first week of the New Year, and she had been out enjoying her time off work. Shelly explained that she had dropped Emma off at our neighbour Nancy's house so that she could play with Nancy's daughter, Emma's best friend. "Perfect timing," I said as I served her a long-necked bottle of Mexican beer from the fridge and sat her at the kitchen table.

For the next half hour I went through each of the bulleted points I had written down. All of them impacted Shelly in some manner. The strategies included who, when, and how to pay for getting a sitter for Emma; the importance of keeping to a routine; the importance of just talking about running; the importance of when I ran; and of course the importance of when and what I ate. I took my time on this point and stressed that there would be no change in this department. I would be eating often and a lot. When I was finished all thirty implementation strategies, I stood up, crumbled the paper into a ball, pushed off backwards from the table, spun on my left leg for a full rotation, and attempted a Toller Cranston liftoff before slamming the paper into the garbage bag.

"What are you doing?" asked Shelly as she placed her hand on the beer bottle to stop it from falling over.

I told her a well-executed single Lutz, of course. She replied that she thought I had stumbled and was about to break my neck on the edge of the stove, reminded me that I didn't have the figure for that move, and then said, "The list, I mean. What are you doing with the list?"

When I told her that its purpose was complete and that it was not to be admired but to be lived, she took one final quick sip of the import and then got up and left the room. The amber refreshment had no cooling effect on the corrosive parting words that burned under her breath.

"I hate New Year's resolutions."

Week 1

Session 1   35 minutes. Run 30 seconds, walk 4 minutes and 30 seconds. Do this 7 times. Tuesday, January 7, 2003

Reporter Jenny Lee's accompanying article to the Document stated that a portion of the Sun Run entry fee would go towards supporting the *Vancouver Sun*'s Raise-a-Reader literacy campaign. According to Jenny, the run was expected to raise $47,000 for Raise-a-Reader that year. I found this interesting because I participate as a reader in Delta's McCloskey Elementary School's Noisy Reading program. Noisy Reading is one of the school's many strategies to raise achievement in primary students' reading comprehension. For Noisy Reading, parents and relatives are encouraged to come to their child's classroom and read to a group of students for half an hour once per week.

When I told my mother about the Noisy Reading program she said, "Oh, I don't read to children at that age." I had no idea what that meant at the time. Was it the voice of experience implying that there was a cut-off point? I'm always mulling something over in my mind, but cut-off points for reading to children had never made the top-million list. Anyway, my mother wouldn't elaborate, knowing I would find out about these things soon enough.

Well, the learning curve was steep. They're a talkative bunch, those little ones. I sat down with about eight of them, and after introducing myself as Emma's dad, I held up the book I was going to read to them. It had looked like a good book when I selected it from the assortment the teacher had placed on the table. It had cute artwork of an animal on the cover, but of more importance it had big letters to read on the inside.

I didn't even get to bring the glossy cover down from over my head before the questions started coming in hard and fast. "Why did it eat my cat?" "Is his cat dead?" "Where do cats go when they're dead?" I was just blown away. I wasn't ready for a discussion group. Really, did Emma get all the kids together before I arrived and warn them that her dad had a preoccupation with death, "So don't talk about it, okay? Oh, and my mama says if he should mention the name Poh-Poh, just nod your head like this, okay?" Poh-Poh would have been a much better representative on the subject of death, but this wasn't ghost story time it was reading time, and Poh-Poh didn't read or write English.

I struggled through that reading session, and as the months went by, I thought I had mastered the group discussion portion of Noisy Reading. Silly me. When the Christmas reading season started, a bombshell landed. With the kids sitting on the schoolroom floor before me, a diminutive voice from the back row sounding as clear as a sleigh bell on a frosty winter's day said, "Santa Claus isn't real you know." Maybe I can be accused of not being properly prepared for these events, but I thought that I was—and probably therein lies the problem. Anyway, there was an immediate and fierce rebuttal from within the group, and after cooling them all down, I could see desperation in their wide eyes as they looked to me for the final word. "Well, I believe in Santa Claus" was my reply, but I felt terrible because the damage could not be undone. I remember exiting the school's heavy double doors to a desolate playground, then putting my head down and not looking forward to Easter.

Late that afternoon, after attaching the Sun Run Document to the fridge and talking to Shelly about my strategy for attaining my goal of fitness, I found myself lying face first on the carpet. The wall-to-wall broadloom smelled as if it could do with a wash and a crusty bit was jabbed into my cheek, but all in all, I felt good. This was session one, week one of my running program, the one with the professional approach. I had just finished my warm-up exercises, the last set consisting of push-ups, and after collapsing I waited for my heart rate to come back down a bit, knowing full well that coming all the way back to normal wasn't possible.

My energy-depleted stare was fixed at one particular nail holding the baseboard to the wall, and I checked whether its nail-set depth was acceptable as I thought back to the *Vancouver Sun*'s Arts and Life section on training for the Sun Run from the day before. Reporter Jenny Lee did a feature on three Greater Vancouver personalities who were training for the Sun Run. The first was a stay-at-home mom named Gwen who was in her forties, had three daughters in elementary school, and claimed she didn't cook, bake, or run. Holy smokes, if she had added that she didn't clean, I would have been spooked—it would have been an exact profile match. Of course, I was rounding off the offspring and the whole gender thing.

The next personality was fun-loving radio host Erin Davis. I remember thinking that Erin was going to be interesting to follow on the *Sun*'s pages over the next thirteen weeks because she was pregnant and also because she was going to walk the Sun Run this year after running it the year before.

Erin's on-air personality was positively vivacious. The problem was that voice. It was out there, but I couldn't figure out where. Reading about her had triggered a memory of some voice-over work Erin had done, but I just couldn't place it. Was it a public service announcement for the Vancouver Airport? Was it the talking moving sidewalk in Los Angles or maybe the talking elevator at the Pan Pacific Hotel? Thanks to Jenny Lee, I now had a new obsession: scanning the airwaves, sound byte by sound byte, for the voice of Erin Davis. Yes, she was out there, but where? This would be a good segue for my years as a sound effects collector, but let's just say I've never been the same since the crows broke me years ago in a misty meadow in Stanley Park and leave it at that.

Jenny featured television morning news anchor Steve Darling next. Over the years I'd seen Steve numerous times in the neighbourhood. Lacing up for a family skate at the Sungod Arena, kicking back at a local coffee house, or even driving by in his car. I heard his name being bandied about by the locals on a regular basis and had seen his name attached to local charity events. But I'd never said hi to him let alone talked to him; I just couldn't stand the embarrassment of exposing myself and all. You know that I'd meet him, then after either drooling or stuttering and possibly even sweating, I'd ask him the important question: "S-so, Steve, d-d-do you know Suzette M-meyers?" Of course he does, but what was he going to be thinking? *Is this guy a crackpot or what? He should be totally captivated by my presence and asking scintillating questions pertaining to the shrine of Steve, not one of my co-workers.* Sorry, Steve, but when it comes to news anchors, Suzette Meyers is stunning and marvellous, and it is she whom I find scintillating. I felt myself melting into the nylon of the cut-pile carpet at the thought of Suzette Meyers and concluded that Steve was a superior choice for the Sun Run feature since I would have been too distracted otherwise.

Steve Darling is a good-looking younger guy who was the sports anchor before sliding over to the news side of the television studio desk. He has an affable personality, and he is *big*. He has a body type like an offensive lineman but without the extra playing weight. Steve looks quite capable of coming out of a three-point stance, say like Jim Mills of B.C. Lions football lore, pulling around the right end with a full head of steam, and laying a licking on you. Of course being the good Canadian kid that he is, I could see Steve doing it gleefully and with a smile.

In the article, Steve said his motivation for Sun Run training was to provide himself with his next fitness challenge. I thought at the time that it sounded as if Steve had a big-picture plan of which the Sun Run was just one component. This intrigued me, and I looked forward to following his progress. After reading about him, I even thought it might be possible to say hi to Steve the next time I saw him. If I did say hi, I figured I would drop the inquiring-minds angle on Suzette Meyers and use the "I have a friend who wants to know" line.

I twisted, turned, and tussled against the forces of gravity that had marooned me in the hallway just outside the bathroom. The struggle turned in my favour when I gained leverage with a grip on the doorway mouldings. I pulled my bulky body up but unintentionally found myself staring into the bathroom mirror. There was a divot in my cheek from the crusty bit on the carpet, and as I began to rub it out I noticed for the first time ever that I could not see my cheekbones or any other skeletal reference points. A ripe, round, and fleshy red face looked back. It occurred to me at that point that I hadn't been to the doctor before starting this whole fitness thing. Apart from the obvious signs of overexertion on my face and the big rolling gut, the rest of my body just seemed swollen.

As I continued to rub my cheek under the vanity lights, I asked myself what Poh-Poh would say about these signs. Would she see them as a warning that I had already exceeded normal operating limits and that I should rest and relax, otherwise I would risk causing irreversible trauma to the body, possibly even death? Poh-Poh was always afraid of tempting the gods. A typical tactic of hers was saying she was going to die in an attempt to trick the gods into thinking they should not waste their time on her and leave her to live another day. Maybe instead of going to the doctor I should use this strategy instead.

I couldn't make up my mind about which way to go; both plans had merits. In that moment of hesitation my feet knew emphatically what to do as they took over and propelled me out of the bathroom, still rubbing my face, before I could pronounce my inevitable demise or make a doctor's appointment.

As I made my way through the hallway towards the back door, I grabbed a denim jacket that I wore when cutting the grass and a stopwatch from the old sound effects days. Within seconds I was running. The house keys were tucked away safe and secure in my jacket pocket as planned, but now I had a different organizational problem. What in the world would I do with this neck strap that seemed like a rope on the stopwatch? My feet kept moving towards the nearest intersection as I fumbled with the non-compliant rope. I can tell you to the exact second how long it took to put this bumbling exercise out of my mind. Fourteen seconds. That's the time that caught my eye during one of the various flip and turn over manoeuvres that I was attempting with my wrist. A wave of panic swept over me. It felt as if I had been running for fourteen minutes, not fourteen seconds, and I wasn't even half finished the first running phase.

My eyes became fixed on the liquid crystal display, which was somewhat easy really because I was now holding the watch about a foot from my face. Although I was counting up to thirty seconds, it was as if I was counting down to destruction, possibly my demise. At twenty seconds I could see blood pooling in my fingertips because of their death grip on the large round casing; within a second more I felt my throat constricting.

During the last nine seconds I held the stopwatch to within inches of my face. My chest had stopped moving as I held my breath, then I held on with a single-minded mission up to the thirty-second mark. I dropped my arm as if my hand had an anvil in its grasp for counterbalance, startled myself with the loudness with which I sucked in some air, and then dared to look around. I saw a spectacular weeping willow tree, and this orientated me to the middle of the intersection just one house down from mine. I remember thinking I should have been much farther, possibly half finished—after all, I felt half dead. Once again, the mesh-panelled babies on my feet didn't stop, and I continued with the four-and-a-half-minute walking portion of the first session.

I spent all of the walking time adjusting the long strap on the stopwatch, checking the time with incessant frequency. Even after I had gotten my gear strapped on and checked it for the proper viewing angle at least a dozen times, I still felt the need to check the time again. This was because I could sense an old passion coming on strong.

Did I ever tell you that I spent most of my adult life working in a manufacturing environment where process control is king? Did you know that to maintain the fundamentals of the process you must measure it on an ongoing basis? Did you know that another reason for measuring is to assess the unequivocal expectation of incremental improvement? Have I ever told you how much I love this Document? I was checking my time so frequently because I had such a high regard for the Document that I did not want to deviate whatsoever from the stated times. I could feel the experience it contained, experience that could be acquired only through scientific analysis of years of trial and error, and I wanted to follow this recipe explicitly. I had an intrinsic belief that this Document—cut out of the newspaper and pasted on another piece of paper and then scribbled upon before being attached to my fridge—would give me the edge required to accomplish my goal of attaining fitness.

But then again, I am an adequate representative of how obsessive compulsive the human species can be. Without question my typing speed is among the world's slowest. The reason is I type with one hand. And why is that? Because my other hand is too busy with a calculator doing word-count projections. I will type a few words, then select Word Count from the Tools drop-down list, then based on the viewed information, calculate a word-count projection (which could be for the paragraph, the page, or the entire manuscript). You may believe as I do that I loved this Document because its systematic approach was familiar territory to me, but when a good dose of reality is factored in, I had simply exchanged my calculator for a stopwatch.

The walking portion of this session took me past the intersection of 112th Street and 80th Avenue. I felt a sense of shame as I walked across the intersection, not because this was where a motorist thought I was committing suicide during my first running initiative—well, yes, that too—but because I was walking. It just didn't feel right to be walking, but I kept my focus and believed in the graduated run/walk process contained in the Document.

I started the second of seven thirty-second runs right after crossing the intersection. Confusion was quick to set in as I soon realized that 80th Avenue became an incline at this point. I had never noticed that before. Sure North Delta rose above Burns Bog and the Fraser River delta via the mighty steep asphalt lanes of Nordel Way, but once you were there I thought it was all pretty flat. The impact on my body was immediate. The stress and strain I had felt during the last ten seconds of the first thirty-second run I was now feeling at the beginning of the second thirty-second run. At the end of this second run, I didn't feel too chipper. I remember looking back over my shoulder at the mountain I had just scaled and almost tossing my stomach contents when I brought my head back around too fast.

The next part of my planned route was to enter the groomed trail around McKitrick Park, which contains the Sungod Recreation Centre, but no way. The eagerness just wasn't there, so I took a shortcut and went down a side street. Of course, there is no such thing as a shortcut when the training session is 100 percent time based, but it sure felt good to think I was taking one. During the much-needed second walking portion of the session, I had two separate instances of elderly gentlemen waving and saying good evening as they passed by. The setting sun did nothing to alleviate my waning enthusiasm as I began to question the wisdom of running farther away from home while it was getting darker with each passing minute. My usual method of operation is to be heading towards home under those circumstances. Thankfully, the gestures of good community spirit soothed my traumatized mind and body and also let me know it was safe outside the comforts of my humble house.

I finished the seven repetitions of session one and essentially staggered into the house, then could not get into the bathtub fast enough after I made one quick phone call. Once out of the tub I got another surprise. Like finding out about inclines in the neighbourhood and being afraid of the dark, I wasn't all that hungry. Oh, well, I didn't dwell on that for long because the pernicious feeling that was at the root of my phone call once again enveloped me in worry. No, I hadn't phoned and left a message for novelist Wayson Choy, with the intention of asking him what his character from the pages of *The Jade Peony* would actually say about my latest ominous health sign. No, I had phoned the Sports and Orthopaedic Physiotherapy Clinic at the Sungod Recreation Centre and made an appointment with the physiotherapist, the real deal. I was in a position of "Danger! Danger! Dave Hutchinson program closedown is imminent!"

Yes, it was true. As much as I had denied it for months, I now had to admit I had a biomechanical weakness. My left heel was throbbing. This was the result after two months of recuperation? After one measly training session my heel had regressed to a position of, at least on the pain threshold scale, being worse than ever. I did not hold the heel in my hands and massage it, ice it, apply heat, or elevate it. Instead I held my face in my hands. It was a crushing moment that drove me to the Internet.

Now, I'm not a big fan of the Internet, and during my first running initiative and up to this point of the Sun Run run/walk program, I hadn't searched once for anything about running, and I thought this was a good thing. There are many reasons for feeling this way, but most of them boil down to trust. The single biggest trust issue was me. I just didn't trust myself, or I should say I didn't trust my ability to interpret the good from the bad from the just plain hoax information that is presented over the Internet. After all, I knew full well that at times, just sometimes, I tended to . . . well, I don't want to say hallucinate, but maybe as Shelly succinctly put it, "Keep dreaming" said it best.

With complete disregard for pain, dejection, and good judgment I marched towards the computer in the kitchen, muttering, "I do not need an operation," over and over again. I felt compelled to do an Internet search because my appointment with the physiotherapist wasn't until Friday. This would be a day after my next planned run, and I couldn't wait that long. I was forced into using my low-speed dial-up connection because I needed information now, but I just needed to keep reminding myself that I did not have to believe everything I read.

A few hours later I knew the theory behind the mechanics of running. I was pleased with this. In my interpretation it was all about energy conservation, and when I coupled this information with the Sun Run Document's strategy of running thirty seconds, I felt there was a positive synchronization of worldwide events taking place.

Unfortunately, I also found out that I needed an operation. I depleted all of that day's remaining common sense to decipher the information being presented to me; it was a mountain of evidence that seemed darn persuasive, in fact gripping at times. Beneath the throbbing of my left heel it felt as if there were two strands of dental floss carving grooves into the bone. I was too afraid to search further and find out how the surgeons would fix this problem, but I imagined it would be similar to the cutting and splicing of a wiring harness, just like in the factory. The more I thought about this, the more I started thinking about the tragic SwissAir airline crash off the east coast near Peggy's Cove a few years back. The leading theory was that it had been caused by a faulty after-market wiring harness. I shut off the computer; put all thoughts of Poh-Poh, SwissAir, and dental floss out of my mind; and vowed that I would not do anything rash—like quitting or even putting off my next training session—until I had a second opinion from the physiotherapist.

Session 2 40 minutes. Run 30 seconds, walk 4 minutes and 30 seconds. Do this 8 times. Thursday, January 9, 2003.

The next morning was the beginning of a non-running day for the program, which I tried to treat with equal importance. I found it quite difficult to get into the rest and relaxation concept. The mind and the body were still ready to move out. After only one training session of the Sun Run program, it was as if the body got a delectable taste of what was to come and wanted more, even with my heel injury. Whereas during my first running initiative of a couple of months earlier, I engorged the body and mind on the process, much like a gluttonous dog feasting on an unattended rump roast. Then like the dog lying on its side gasping, puking, and unable to walk, the voracious need for more had been removed, however temporarily. Anyway this excess energy was easy to spot, mainly because I hadn't felt this way in years. After wondering what to do with myself, I decided to go swimming at the Sungod Recreation Centre, but that would be in the afternoon. That morning I had other plans.

The fact that I hadn't gone to the doctor before starting such a physical endeavour made me uncomfortable to the point of feeling that I may have been encouraging calamity to strike. You can believe it or not, but I was not in the same league as Poh-Poh when it came to these matters. In addition, it was not like me to throw caution to the wind when it came to safety. Prudence was once again in the ripped and stuffing-oozing driver's seat as I made my way to the local drugstore. Time was of the essence, and I just couldn't get to my family doctor fast enough; the blood pressure machine would have to suffice.

I checked my blood pressure once, then walked around the drugstore before checking a second time. Of course I felt all hot and bothered and unbelievably guilty as I sauntered around the aisles waiting to do the second blood pressure check, knowing that the shoplifting detectives with their cameras and all were watching my every move. I was tempted to cruise the aisles with my hands above my head declaring my innocence, but I figured that would skew the tests.

During the second pump-and-squeeze session I checked the machine for a calibration sticker. I didn't find one, so after the second reading I got back in the car and drove to another drugstore to use their blood pressure testing equipment. In total I went to three different drugstores that morning, with all three informing me that my blood pressure was, dare I say it, normal. Oh, I knew that; I was just testing the equipment for, you know, uniformity, compliance, and hygiene issues.

Swimming later that day was great. The indoor pool at the Sungod Recreation Centre in McKitrick Park had undergone a major renovation and had been reopened for only a few months. The old pool had been expanded to include a heated training pool for young beginners and a heated recreational pool for young tots, which included a forced-water section called the River. The eight million dollar renovation also included a steam room, a sauna, a hot tub, and a new lap section called the Sunshine Pool, where swimming competitions could be held.

The Sunshine Pool and most of the other newly built amenities were housed under a large arched roof featuring gorgeous laminated wood support beams that gleamed brilliantly in the reflected light from the pool. This architectural statement greets you at the front entranceway, then with its appealing lines it draws your eye to an overview of the entire facility, where there are six other beams of the same striking design. At least I hope that was where everyone's eyes were. Wearing a bathing suit when you have an overhang is just plain rough.

The outside walls of the Sunshine Pool were floor-to-ceiling windows that bathed the area in natural light, hence the pool's name. While I burned off my excess energy in the pool and then again while I walked the short distance back home, I psyched myself up for the next day's training session. I knew that at the end of the week the physiotherapist might order me to fold the Document and shut the program down. Until such time, though, I had developed a bulldozer mentality wherein I was prepared .to plow through the safe and comforting confines of home and leave it all on the street, hopefully not under some vehicle.

While doing my stretching exercises before the second training session, I did not want to dwell on my heel injury, so I concentrated on all the positive aspects that had taken place up to this point. My denim lawnmower jacket was working out just fine. It was lightweight, loose fitting, and best of all it zipped up to the chin. This allowed me to build up some body heat at the beginning of the run, then I could release it as both heat and perspiration accumulated. The typical January temperature in the Greater Vancouver area was just above zero Celsius. The sweatpants were unlined, and I remember thinking that they were just perfect and how could I have made such an intelligent retail purchase. Of course, I later remembered that Shelly had given them to me as a Christmas present years ago. The long-sleeved T-shirt and socks weren't causing any problems, and as for the stopwatch, once I had the darn rope wrapped around my hand without cutting off the circulation, I found it to be proficient. In fact, the functionality of the large digital numbers on the display was quite alluring.

How about those shoes? Well, the shoes were smooth operators. The mesh-panelled babies made me feel as if I were part of a machine. Oh, they were good. The first training session may have been a physically imposing challenge, but I completed it and I had to give the shoes some credit. They did a wonderful job of being the mediator between the brute force and ignorance of my willpower and the hard surface of the road. They gave me a sense of control and stability, which brought the sure-footed factor way up to the highest percentile. The lightweight design coupled with the cool winter breeze blowing over the balls of my feet gave me the impression that I was running with only a sophisticated membrane attached to my soles. The mesh-panelled babies relayed messages from the road that were intriguing if not downright seductive. The signal back said, *Go*. With each step the mesh-panelled babies were saying, *It's all right, push harder, use more force, test me, use me, take me to a higher level.* If only I could—okay, yes, I promise . . . yes, yes, yes, we will fly. They were that good, the best I'd ever had.

By far the most positive aspect up to this point was my attitude. I wasn't having a problem at all getting out the door; coming back in was a different story. I must admit at the time that I was more than a bit surprised at my enthusiasm for this project. But in looking back I think the main reason was the high level of interest. Overall, the training program had a grip on me.

First off there was the Document, which had secured my entry and now had me willing to raise the ante. The Document even had the smell of being the real McCoy. Then there was *Vancouver Sun* reporter Jenny Lee's feature article. It had a crisp certainty in its quality that instilled confidence in this reader. The three runners selected to highlight and promote the training program had varied backgrounds, with their individual takes on the program all coming across as genuine. From the get-go I wanted to know how their personal Sun Run stories would end.

The program and the feature writing had all of this to interest me and more. How much more could there be? Well, I didn't have a big windmill moment where the dog almost became a victim of my delight, but I did laugh aloud and startle the children in the street when I read a certain name. Buried in the middle portion of Jenny Lee's feature article, and the only mention of it in three full newsprint pages pertaining to the Sun Run, was the *Vancouver Sun*'s purveyor of opinions, columnist Pete McMartin. To me this was above-the-fold, front page headline news. The understatement of Pete McMartin's contribution as a participant in that year's Sun Run was truly a conservative cards-to-the-vest approach. The Pete McMartin card—of course it's wild—would be played the following week in the first of his weekly columns on his Sun Run training experiences.

I finished off the stretching exercises, and as I started down the street, I was trying to figure out if my diminished hunger the last couple of days should be filed under a positive aspect of the training program or as one of Poh-Poh's signs of an imminent health crisis. The filing was swept aside once I hit the gradual incline on 80th Avenue just past the supposed dive-of-death corner. I kept looking over my shoulder on the incline just to see if it looked steeper from the opposite angle. This was crazy; I was taxing all my reserves at the beginning of the training session. All this effort just to make it up an incline that I had never even considered an incline or any other version of a grade up to this point, and I had driven past it every single day for more than four years.

Whether it was the overgrown foliage, the constant looking over my shoulder, the vista of Burns Bog at the top of the incline, or the peripheral blindness brought on from sheer exhaustion, I missed the trail leading into the park. Emma calls this trailhead the secret entrance to the park. There is no signage or any other form of invitation other than a small opening in a thicket of underbrush and trees. I took one last look at the Burns Bog vista and was in awe of its astonishing lack of human encroachment—there is nary a shingle to be seen—then I turned and started back for the secret entrance.

Once I was through the trailhead, some bramble bushes made multiple lassoing attempts to attach themselves to my sweatpants. The barbed bushes couldn't slow me down, though, because I didn't think I could go any slower. I was running with the paranoia of further injury set to maximum, and to tell you the truth, I felt comfortable doing this. My compliance with the Internet running instructions was just slightly exaggerated, with the result being reduced speed. I did not lock my knees so that I could get them under me, allowing them to act as the shock absorbers they were meant to be. I also kept the strides much shorter on that day to minimize the impact on my left heel. My Internet research also said not to use the toe or the heel as primary areas of landing since these areas were for sprinting, not distance running. This all suited me just fine, but because it did, I wondered if I was using selected information to bolster any preconceived notions of running.

Within a minute the barbed gauntlet ended, and I came upon the groomed running trail of McKitrick Park. Even though I was in the walking portion of the training session at this time, I remember the soft, cushiony feel of the trail underneath the mesh-panelled babies. I knew then that I would make it through that day's session; up until then, lurking in the deepest, darkest regions of my mind, was a feeling that my heel could give out at any time.

The walking portion felt strange; after I caught my breath from the running portion, it was actually a long, leisurely time of doing nothing. I didn't stride it out during the walking portions, either. I put them to good use in my quest for survival by using them to conserve as much energy as possible until the next thirty-second session. It wasn't long before my mind filled this seemingly empty portion of the training with thoughts of something seemingly important, like Pete McMartin's involvement in all this.

To succinctly capture what Pete McMartin was all about, I needed only to recall a letter to the editor about him from a few years back. No, I didn't write it, nor did I have a friend of a friend write it. I don't even know what the letter was all about, and I didn't have it cut out, pasted up, and saved on the fridge like the Sun Run training Document, so I can't repeat it verbatim. I don't even think the letter writer knew what it was really about, either, because all he did throughout the letter was rant about McMartin's picture at the top of his column. What type of man would take the time to write a letter to the editor of a major newspaper and then go on and on about what a columnist looked like? I mean, we could all see for ourselves at the bottom of section B that he looked (dare I say it?) rather handsome.

Getting back to what kind of man would write a letter slamming McMartin's physical features, well an angry, fed-up-to-here man who just wasn't going to take it anymore. A man who had been forced to the brink of who knows where but while on this obviously slippery slope had lost his ability to form a reasonable rebuttal. Pete McMartin evoked over-the-top emotive qualities in that letter writer, but McMartin's penchant for provocative and free-wheeling columns leave all his readers susceptible to some form of involuntary reaction. The emotional states of these reactions were as varied as McMartin's ability to convey them in his cleverly constructed columns, where often his hilarity was matched by his ability to infuriate the reader. Pete McMartin could make you laugh, cry, or attack his very image.

I just couldn't imagine someone taking the same umbrage with Jenny Lee as was taken with McMartin. She is a young mother with an engaging smile who writes for the Healthy Life section in the *Vancouver Sun* newspaper. I mean, who could get all worked up about Jenny after, say, her work just before Christmas of that year? In her article she pitched tips on how to combat Christmas stress by eating high-quality dark chocolate. Wow, doesn't that make you want to pick up a pen and rip Jenny's latest hairstyle?

Speaking of style, what about McMartin's? His picture, by the way, was of a Caucasian man in his late forties with a thick-seeded, dark-coloured hairline. He had chubby cheeks and a sardonic smirk, let's just say like Dennis the Menace would have if the fictional character were allowed to grow up. I didn't know if McMartin's style had grace—I'd never met the man—but they say pictures have an extraordinary word-count value, and while his picture was uncommitted on grace, it did say that he had panache.

The cropping of the picture at the top of his column showed an unbuttoned shirt collar, with some sort of unidentifiable fashion accessory hung loose around his neck. The easy bet would be that the accessory was a tie, but this was Pete McMartin and one should scrutinize the exposed cards just a tad closer. After all, in previous pictures since 1976, the year he began his career at the *Vancouver Sun*, he had on at least one occasion shown up for the photo shoot wearing suspenders and a bow tie. So based on the eclecticism of his past fashion behaviour, and of course from years of immersing myself in the local culture, I felt with about 99 percent certainty that the man had taken up local author Stanley Coren's fashionista custom of wearing a scarf, McMartin's twist being the knot versus the ring. The remaining 1 percent was for wriggle room on the outside chance he was wearing whatever it is that Canadian lawyers and judges wear as neckpieces. You know, the more I thought about it, the more I wanted to decrease that wriggle room.

I had perfect timing as I finished the eighth and final walking repetition at the back door of my house. The second session was an interminable five minutes longer than the first session, or at least the run/walk time was five minutes longer. For the actual total training session time I included the pre-run exercise time and the post-run shower time, which ended up being ninety-nine minutes. Making the training session time as short as possible was one of my implementation strategies. I had identified an overly long total training time as a potential point-of-process failure. I didn't want to dilly-dally around and then end up stretching out the pain and misery. Intense, short, and sweet was the motto, and then get on with something else. For this reason I kept the stopwatch going, and it wasn't until I was showered and dressed that I stopped the watch and began the reflection process. Ninety-nine minutes? I could knock that down some, mostly in the showering and dressing time.

At that point I felt I needed to keep an overly long exercise time, if for anything just to have the extra time to work on the motivational aspects of the training. So far I liked the fact that I had been able to go out the door all pumped up and ready for action. The total time was within the forecasted nominal range (and that was good), but my heel hurt (and that was not good). I had some huge compensatory activity going on, especially with the shorter strides. This got me through the session, but I had a feeling of impending doom as I thought ahead to the physiotherapy appointment scheduled for the next day.

I had another problem—well, maybe just a concern—but this whole running program had left me exhausted. It felt as if I was getting a bit feverish, like maybe coming down with the flu and my body was slowly shutting down. Funny thing was, in the feed a fever, starve a cold adage I wasn't all that hungry. I finished off that day's reflective portion of the training session by attempting to get all thoughts of my heel, my surgery, and all things Poh-Poh off my mind by taking Rosie for a walk. I furthered the disassociative process by thinking about McMartin's scarf. I remember mulling over the geographical equation regarding McMartin's fashion sense during his youth. I concluded the walk with the realization that I didn't have the foggiest notion of what in the world really goes on in that distant land of southern Ontario.

Session 3   40 minutes. Run 30 seconds, walk 4 minutes and 30 seconds. Do this 8 times. Sunday, January 12, 2003.

The next day I walked Emma to school and on the way back continued past the house and on towards the Sungod Recreation Centre in McKitrick Park for my appointment. Even on my rest days I was trying to do as much walking outside as possible. I thought of it as acclimatizing or even conditioning myself through a bit of cross-training. I was a little suspicious that the soles of my feet might not be up to the rigours of this whole training thing (you know, blisters and whatnot), plus I wanted to get used to being out and about in the rain for long periods of time. Now I'd done my fair share of standing out in the rain over the last couple of years watching Emma play soccer, but that had been just a once-a-week type of thing. The Document said I needed to be out in the elements three times a week, and it wasn't my intention to be a fair-weather runner. I planned to go rain or shine. This was Greater Vancouver after all, and the ability to play outside every day of the year is legendary.

I unfortunately arrived on time as usual. I envy people who can be late. The receptionist directed me to a chair in the reception area after we dealt with some administrative details, like paying for all this. I remember sitting down and thinking it just didn't seem right that one should have to pay for bad news. Of course I was being presumptuous at this point, but I could feel a retail situation coming on as I sat there, and I didn't like it one iota. If it was just like a retail situation, should I renegotiate after getting the bad news—you know, like getting a deal at a scratch-and-dent sale? I wasn't sure what to do, but just thinking about the possibility of adding to a long line of poorly executed retail transactions increased my already high anxiety. Oh, I needed relief, and I found it, shock of all shocks, at the end of two dark tunnels.

Since I had unpredictably found myself feeling as if I were in a retail environment, I was searching the document-laden walls, the tan brown medical files with their dashes of colour, and the standard white drop ceiling for the inevitable closed-circuit television cameras. It was then that I spotted the viscous nasal passages of some young lad, his face pressed up against the physiotherapist's window for my exclusive viewing. I could see him but not hear him; he was walking out of the swimming pool corridor with a group of equally young and rambunctious friends. It was a quick press and glide, exposing a white pig's nose on slime before he exited the automatic doors.

After my victimization, I took back my first notion of the recreation centre's complex smells and furthered the categorization process. When I had first sat down I thought I smelled new paint, drywall, carpet, and other construction aromas associated with a major renovation mingling with the pool's chlorine and high humidity. The physiotherapist's offices and treatment facilities were a new addition to the Sungod Recreation Centre, along with a new gym, an aerobic and dance studio, and a weight room. The adjoining ice rink got a new floor as well. Now I'm a guy who is used to industrial strength applications after putting in some years at the factory, but after watching the smear and run tactics of this kid, I didn't need to guess that interior designers have a heavy-duty aspect to their jobs as well. At least I hoped they did or this facility wasn't going to go the distance.

The receptionist called me and walked me through an exercise area to an examination room. Once inside, she handed me a pair of workout shorts and instructed me to put them on. I was surprised by this, but I guess it was better than a gown, or even worse she could have handed me a container and asked for a sample. I was sure all of that would come at a later date. I hadn't finished surveying the examination room before the physiotherapist slipped in. He was a tall young man who wore an expression of concern, like someone who had just heard on the radio that the restaurant where he ate last night had just issued a hepatitis warning. I felt reassured by his demeanour.

We introduced ourselves, then he told me I hadn't needed to put my shoes back on. As I unlaced the footwear, I unloaded the medical history of my left heel over the last two months, including the information that my fascia was embedded in my heel. I didn't get a response to my medical viewpoint, which I took as a sign of how serious the situation was. He could probably sense, maybe even see, the problem already.

Before I knew it I was like the kid from the reception area; the physiotherapist had me turned with my nose up to the wall as he poked and prodded the entire length of my backside from the top of my head to the bottom of my feet. During these deep forefinger and thumb probes, I felt that one rib in particular was taken way beyond its stated compression tolerance. When I finished my mercy seeking moan the physiotherapist mentioned that I should have worn my runners, whose condition would have given him a greater insight into my situation.

Keeping my nose to the wall, I cast my eyes down to the high-gloss black oxfords. Oh, I must have looked like a dork standing there in the grey workout shorts with my tucked-in, crisply pressed, button-down shirt and the just-polished-that-morning shoes on. It got worse the longer I stared at them. Besides the strain of having my eyes at such an unnatural angle, I began fretting about whether the physiotherapist knew they were steel-toed as well, which would have only heightened the embarrassment. Just what had I been thinking, that a medicine ball was going to run over my toes? And just what other dangers had I been preparing myself for, dropped dumb bells? I was working out all of this overprotectiveness when I heard, "Excuse me. . . . *Excuse me. . . . Now, tell me why you think your injury is so serious.*"

I delved into my story of not wanting to go on the Internet but doing so anyway and that surgery was what I concluded to be the only rational outcome. I wanted to ask him his truthful opinion of my chances for a full recovery, but he had me do a pirouette and a small jump, then he laid me flat out on my back on the examination table before I could inquire. His muscular hands soon had my legs in a forward backward open scissors position as he forced himself upon my hamstrings. I caught a glimpse of his brow through my stretched-out appendages; it appeared deeply furrowed. At the time I thought it to be the look of a man who had become encased in deep empathy. It never occurred to me that it could be the expression of extreme physical exertion.

He then asked about the condition of my back. This is where I took the opposite tact from Poh-Poh. Whereas she would have openly talked about her impending death, I on the other hand didn't want to disturb the bad-back spirits, and my reply contained as few words as possible. Besides I was out of breath, what with all this unnatural and involuntary exercise being forced upon my body. My reply was honest, though, and I told him that my back felt the best it had in years. This is what made my heel injury so frustrating. It was my back that was supposed to be my Achilles heel, if you know what I mean.

I had injured my back during a pick-up game of football in the early eighties. I guess in the long term it was life altering, but at the time it was pretty innocent stuff. It all went down during an Indian summer under a brilliant blue sky on a vacant double-wide Kitsilano lot. I realize the chances of those three circumstances coinciding again in Greater Vancouver are remote, but they did take place. I had just completed your basic high-speed fake and shake before I turned and looked for the ball. I was expecting the ball's spiral trajectory to be dialed in on my black-haired shirt but it was woefully underthrown and heading for the darkness of the dirt.

What happened next is something that a receiver, regardless of sport, has almost no control over. A blend of instinct, competitiveness, athleticism, and years of practice while growing up triggered the fast-twitch muscles, and I bent over and made the catch off my shoelaces. It wasn't really a big deal. There was no euphoria of having done something special. It was just done and you played on, but this time I did feel a small twinge in my back.

Well, the small twinge turned into years of health problems with my back. Eventually I got better, but I never really bounced all the way back. Normal everyday living was fine, but I found that my back had become a weak link, and being physically competitive was out of the question. I just couldn't burn. I didn't want to get into any of this with the physiotherapist since my back was truly not causing me problems—well, no major problems, anyway—plus I didn't have the audacity of Poh-Poh to tempt fate.

Now I didn't bring up this whole back issue so that I could brag about my former athletic prowess, and before you think I used to be a runner of some esteem who just needed a bit of a tune-up, consider these three points. First off, receivers sprint. This equates to small distances, which I've always found appealing, especially the ten-yard buttonhook. Second off, and this is very important, there were no touchdown dances, ever. Third off, I was a legend in my own mind. Have I ever told you about my golden cleats?

After our short talk on the condition of my back, the physiotherapist had me slide off the table and put my nose up against the wall again. This time he asked me to stand on some sort of angled exercise device that positioned the backs of my heels to the ground and forced my toes to point upward to my chin. I felt some strain in the lower backs of my legs. The physiotherapist told me that my calf muscles needed to be worked on several times a day. He went on about how to exercise them without his exercise device and handed me a few sheets of paper containing diagrams. He then mentioned that he would be talking to the Sun Run clinic operating out of the Sungod Recreation Centre.

I found it all interesting, but what about me? What about the surgery? I could feel the session closing, and I pushed myself to ask about the medical procedure on my left heel. A frown accentuated all the lines on his face as he said, "Stretch it." That was it, stretch it. The weight of the exercise papers became too much as I let my arm fall to my side, not giving a darn if I gave myself a paper cut on my exposed thigh. I then exhaled long and hard before turning to retrieve my clothing.

You would think I would be happy not to be condemned to going under the knife, but I was mortified. Was that it, a few simple exercises? I felt shame at the simplicity of it all, then humiliation when I bent over to pick up my industrial-strength dress shoes. Of course I mumbled a thank you to him as I walked out the office door with hunched shoulders. The last words of his reply were, "Come back in two weeks if it's not better."

I strained under the weight of the walk home. The truth that emanated from the Sungod offices was not only a burden but also striking in its clarity. He was right. Of all the exercises I was doing, not one dealt with my calf muscles. It was a deplorable revelation, it was a crucial oversight of a major muscle group, it was downright dim. I again reviewed my learned fundamentals of exercise from the Trudeau-era fitness initiative from the seventies. By the time I had walked home, then slogged through the overgrown grass in the backyard on my way to the storage shed, I had concluded that it was just a case of if you don't use it, you lose it. I had been away from a lifestyle that included physical fitness for far too long, at least that was the most generous reason I could come up with.

I fumbled my way out of the shed carrying a piece of half-inch plywood, a two by four offcut, screws, a handsaw, and a speed square. The power tools I kept in the house. No, I wasn't boldly disregarding professional advice and building a leg splint, I was fabricating one of those new-fangled calf-stretching devices. Well, it was new to me.

I custom cut all the pieces so that the device would fit into a corner in the kitchen, then I screwed it together. My intention was to have it accessible and ready for action at all times; you know, while drying the dishes I could get in a little stretch time. The big selling point on Shelly's having this pile of wood permanently in her kitchen would be, "This device will cut towel snapping by 50 percent." I was sure she would go for it. If I could somehow verify my math, she probably would demand a matching set. I introduced the device to the family later that night at a craft party. We all traced an outline of one of our feet on the front of the device, including Rosie, then Emma painted it.

Two days later I found myself on another mission: Operation Weigh-In. There are many reasons why an elderly woman who has been wheelchair bound since early childhood would have a bathroom scale, and I'm one of them. My cousin Helen has lovely flowing white hair, pillow-soft cheeks that are cushioned from within by the kindest of souls and a personality that outmatches in both size and warmth the substantial stone fireplace she usually wheels herself next to. Of course, she also has the scale.

It was not even a week into the Sun Run training program and I was already having trouble with my goals, objective statements, and whatnot. Yes, the weight issue had raised its ugly head once again, probably the minute my surgery was taken off the table. It was Sunday, and I had the family in Shelly's SUV, including the dog, heading into Vancouver to visit cousin Helen. It was a serious mission; my hands were gripped tight on the wheel, I was assertive in reaching the speed limit, and I was cutting out the usual celebrity/movie star sightseeing banter, with the exception of hockey player Markus Naslund's house. Pretty much every trip to cousin Helen's, Emma insisted that I point out the house of the Vancouver Canucks captain.

Once we were inside Helen's, I pushed the borders of rudeness and headed straight for the scale. We didn't have a scale in Delta. There were many other accessories that we also didn't have, like a "home sweet home" embroidered wall hanging. I lifted a plastic-bag-lined wastepaper basket off the scale, then pulled it from its corner along the bare bathroom floor. It's all-metal casing made a heavy flat sound throughout this dragging stage, then it gave another distinctive clang as I dropped the lifted end into position. My eyes verified the authenticity of the scale by first examining the dark irregular splotches of rust on the edges of the white metal rotary wheel, then the familiar large black numbers. I didn't need to calibrate this instrument with any plus-five or minus-five hooey—it spoke the truth and had since I first started using it around the hundred pound mark.

I placed my feet on the scale with the accompanying sound of scratched paper and a slight tickling sensation on the bottom of my socks. The decorative paper veneer where the feet were placed had begun to curl on the edges, but I was confident that its accuracy hadn't been compromised. I usually weigh myself at cousin Helen's once, maybe twice a year. I woke up that morning with the sinking feeling that if I didn't get to Helen's as soon as possible, too many training sessions would go by, and I would have lost an opportunity for some realistic benchmarking on the weight side of things. I couldn't remember the last time I had weighed myself, and I had no idea how much I weighed other than just too darn much. The numbers rolled to the right, then swung back with equal velocity on the first of about five swings. The wild swings got shorter and shorter until they became gentle rocks, then they stopped and the truth was revealed. Two hundred and twenty pounds. Mission accomplished.

My socked feet padded across the hardwood floor to the sofa opposite the fireplace, where I mulled over this new-found knowledge and did not join in the conversation—well, at least I didn't join wholeheartedly. I had other things on my mind, such as how much I should really weigh. I couldn't use the Internet to figure it out since I had promised myself after leaving the physiotherapist's that there would be no more medical-related searches for the remainder of the Sun Run program. My biggest fear that day at Helen's was breaking my no Internet promise, then taking an avid interest in some wacko site, maybe titled "Weight Loss through Self-Surgery." By the end of the visit I concluded that I would weigh myself once more after running the Sun Run—just for curiosity's sake, right? Since I had no idea how much I should weigh, I used my weight of one hundred and sixty pounds from eight years earlier to get the goalposts of my mind-map properly aligned.

Let's see now, this Sun Run program was forcing me to review and put into context a few things I didn't usually consider over the course of a normal day. Stuff like how I quit exercising twenty years ago, quit speeding fifteen years ago, quit drinking ten years ago, quit smoking eight years ago, quit flying last year, quit the Internet on Friday.

An endeavour of my mother's many years ago was to teach me that an attempt to improve myself by removing my flaws was not necessarily going to result in my becoming a better person. She used the example of my dad quitting drinking as her prime case in point. She would always say that his quitting never brought about real change and that I should take note of this. Evidently, from reviewing my quit list, with its duration of time and diversity of subject matter, I'm a lousy note taker and I failed this life lesson. In fact the mode of failure was so utterly complete that I was now running out of things to quit, so I had to create something new to quit, and that I did. A big, round, hairy, and pasty-white sixty-pound belly that didn't jiggle, it moved in tsunami waves. Of course, weight loss was not a Sun Run goal. In retrospect, not only was the weather hard during those early years I spent growing up on the windswept prairies, so was the learning.

That Sunday evening I extended my recovery time between the second and third training sessions of week one to more than three full days by running as late as I could. Even with the thirty-second running portions, the incline on 80th Avenue just after 112th Street was pushing my boundaries of physical ability. It truly felt as if I were going to pop a blood vessel. It was too much, and on top of all that, because it was so early in the training session, it put a damper on the rest of my outing in the park.

The four and a half minutes of walking time was spent studying the mechanics of my foot hitting the soft ground of the trail that encompassed the perimeter of McKitrick Park. That and practicing some sort of quick-reflex martial arts move where my hand moved in lightning fashion from my waist to within inches of my face every fifteen seconds. I had an unquenchable need to know the time left in the repetition . . . under less than ideal lighting conditions . . . using the stopwatch that did not have a backlight feature. My experience in the two previous training sessions where I had used the stopwatch in a carrot-on-a-stick fashion had left me pondering whether a little Toller Cranston choreography would enhance this process. But with the invention of this new move performed in the dark shadows of the tall trees in the park, I would need to start wearing a helmet and face guard if I didn't put some flair and finesse into the manoeuvre sooner rather than later.

After studying my feet and left hand, I moved on to the rest of my body. I was looking for ways to conserve energy. The short strides I was using to protect my left heel, when coupled with a concentrated effort to keep my shoulders loose and my chin up, produced an energy-efficient stride. During about the third walking repetition, I came to a stunning energy-saving conclusion: I needed a different route to the park.

The Document's stated requirements of week one ended with an impeccably timed session-ending entrance through the back door of the house, where I went straight to the painted pile of wood and got in a little stretch time before collapsing at the kitchen table.

The front door opened, and Shelly breezed in with the child in tow and the apricot hues of Rosie snuggled in a precious two-armed cradle fashioned out of Shelly's loose beige wool sweater. My wife started to chat the second the door opened but stopped after I gave her some man-in-dire-circumstances hand signals. I was having trouble hearing between all the gasping and everything, plus I couldn't comprehend what little I did hear. Finally, after about five *whats*, I got to the bottom of the story. Pete McMartin would probably have needed only one perfectly mouthed lip-reader's *what*. You see, my *whats* were incomplete, sort of like the thinly sliced Swiss cheese of *whats*, with their holes and everything. McMartin's *whats* would be like a big block of aged marbled cheddar, heavy stuff combined with low stink.

Shelly, who is *what* and lactose tolerant by the way, was returning from a visit with our neighbour and said that Emma's best friend's mom had joined the Sun Run training clinic, which was starting tomorrow. This information acted like smelling salts on me, and it didn't take long before I was up pacing the kitchen while hand-combing my thinning hair and introducing a fresh volley of *whats*. I was shocked by our neighbour Nancy's involvement. Not by the fact that she was doing it—she was a young, vibrant woman in good health and more than capable—no, I was shocked that anyone I knew was doing the exact same program I was doing at precisely the same time, on the same street. I hadn't taken this variable into account.

My mind reeled while my head rolled and the appliances attained liftoff. Oh, the pressure, such insufferable pressure. I could feel a round of chocolate-dipped doughnuts coming on strong. I blurted my biggest and loudest *what* of the night, which elicited a small growl from the dog being held in Shelly's bosom, when she said that Nancy was going to be a Vancouver Sun Run Team Leader.

Week 2

Session 1 45 minutes. Run 1 minute, walk 4 minutes. Do this 9 times. Tuesday, January 14, 2003.

The unease of week two started the moment I opened my eyes and tossed aside the pillow that kept me from seeing the textured ceiling. I had been tossing and turning most of the night, working on a new route to the park. In typical fashion I had made a mountain out of a molehill. After all, there were only two straightforward options of getting to the park from my house. Well, actually three if not using the trail in McKitrick Park was an option. Unfortunately, I did give option three a good portion of the sleepless night before disregarding it. In the end I figured the Sungod Track, as I had renamed it, was the key to my success in reaching my goal of attaining fitness by completing the Sun Run program.

Intrinsically, I felt my biggest obstacle to attaining this goal was going to be a weight-related problem. I believed the now disproportional amount of weight being placed on my joints would result in a lower body injury of some sort. I've seen it many times over the years (remember, I was doing more watching than doing)—older men taking their Volkswagen bodies to the ski slopes or down the concrete sidewalks and pushing them to perform like Porsches. Lots of broken arms, busted backs, sprained ankles, and bruised egos, but the most common result was blown knees.

Hey, I'll admit it, I have a low pain threshold. I'm just not going there, plus I like living in a calm, soothing environment. It's a care and maintenance of the central nervous system type of thing. Shelly pretty much threatens primal scream therapy whenever I moan and groan, and if I were to add crutches to that scenario I'm sure it would be like introducing not one but two command signals for the execution of the violent home remedy. So the Sungod Track, with its soft bark-mulch trail, was in—big time.

The plan was to use the trail, which would go easy on my knees until I either lost weight or got my legs in shape, then I would take myself out on a concrete tour. It was the no-scream component of my implementation strategies. You know, the ones I tossed in the garbage, which included the gentle ambience of running in the greenery of the park and being comforted by the fact that its benefits would extend beyond the track to the sanity of my household and the neighbouring households. The only problem was how to get there.

After additional time spent tossing and turning, I finally figured out why I had originally chosen the longer of the two routes to the Sungod Track: I didn't want Audrey and Ted to see me. Oh, this is a narcissistic beauty. Audrey and Ted live on the short, flat route to the track, and they both worked at the same factory I did before I was laid off. In fact, Audrey worked in the same department I did and was laid off on the same day I was. Ted left the factory of his own accord a few weeks later after finding another job. A young couple without children, they had purchased a house in the area the previous year. Of course I used to talk to Audrey on a daily basis, and we'd talked since we were laid off. I do know her and all, but that didn't mean she needed to see me in all my meekness walking by her house.

The way I had it figured, the thirty-second running portion of last week's sessions would have taken me to just before their house. This week's one-minute running portion of the session would have me stop pretty much at the foot of their driveway in a full blather of sweat and a bluster of exhaustion. It wasn't as if going a little bit farther was an option; on that morning I figured I'd be lucky if I made the one-minute mark without stopping. The worst part about this whole dishonour of stopping running wouldn't have been the debasement of my image by fighting for air or the disgrace of an inglorious walk-by of their house. No, the worst part would have been the prolongation of the assault on my vanity. You see, they lived on a large corner lot that sat on the two streets I needed to take for the shorter route to the Sungod Track.

My final bedtime decision to take the shorter way was based on a simple principle of life or death. Thankfully I didn't use any Poh-Poh strategies, and I chose self-preservation, but not without recalling the training Document's contents and projecting weeks of anguish before I would be able to run with the utter nonchalance and ease of stride of a trained athlete past Audrey and Ted's corner lot. Yes, the theatre of my mind had some serious image projection happening, but it did bring me tranquility and eventual sleep.

The next morning I was bursting with energy, not knowing whether I could complete the one-minute run portion, which had me going great guns down the driveway instead of my usual start once I hit the road. Then of course there was the ambiguity of the corner lot to contend with. I made a hard left at the willow tree, and then a queer sense of accomplishment washed over me when I transitioned from running to walking, in one step. Yes, I had made the one-minute mark, and yes, my late-night time and distance projections had been correct: I had stopped running with complete accuracy in front of Audrey and Ted's driveway. I got off easy that morning because their blinds were closed as tight as my constricted windpipe. I was on the Sungod Track during the first walking repetition and feeling good about keeping to the Document, or maybe I should admit that the lack of any early inclines or voyeurs had put me in a proper frame of mind.

Speaking of voyeurs, the looky-loo aspect or lack of it was another great feature of training on the Sungod Track. With its trail weaving its way in and out of the mostly forty-foot-tall alder trees and then looping behind the Sungod Pool and Sungod Ice Rink facilities, it was very difficult to get a good look at any of its users for any length of time. The looped trail was L-shaped, with the top of the L oriented to the north. The unassuming secret entrance was at the top of the L, where I entered during week one off 80th Avenue.

Starting this day in week two, I entered from the starboard side of the L, or its east entrance off 112th Street and 78th Avenue, where six good-sized rocks were laid out like a fallen inukshuk for guidance. I found this visual cue stuff important since my ability to process visual information was degraded under the extreme physical exertion demanded by the Document, what with all the sweat streaming into my eyes, steamed glasses, bouncing eyeballs, general jostling of the brain, and of course operating the stopwatch. This made the Sungod Track all the more appealing. After only one week it had already become a sanctuary, a safe haven away from motor vehicles, hard running surfaces, and if the truth be known, the looky-loos. Whether it was team sports or just my many years of being involved in a team environment at work, I looked forward to the new experience of the individual challenge and the isolation of the track, with its quiet and safe setting enhancing this quest. Plus, let's say if I had joined a Sun Run clinic, there was something profoundly disturbing in exposing the gutter-dwelling extent of your human frailty to a group of people let alone to the first-impression scrutiny of a single person whom you do not know.

I could feel a sharp, cold spike of pain in my left heel with each ground strike, whether I was walking or running. It was as if the heel had balled up the ninety-eight degree dental floss, and after disposing it in the nearest fluid flow, exchanged it for some sub-zero nitrogen-cooled dental floss. Based on this negative cause and effect, my running form became a point of fixation. Then as the minutes accumulated in the training session, I focused on my heel. The stretching had made a big improvement, so much so that I now felt I had a chance at continuing the training, but I had no idea how long I would need to endure the pain.

It was out of fear that I would overwhelm myself with worry by appraising each left foot plant that I forced myself to switch mental gears. If I hadn't switched gears, I could see myself standing somewhere on the Sungod Track with my left foot just hanging in the air. I would not be running, I would just be standing mid-trail, mid-stride and thinking about running. Believe me this was more than possible, so I did a mental switch and moved on.

Pete McMartin's mug and his dangly scarf were next on my mind. McMartin's first column for this year's Sun Run had been yesterday, and it was exactly as I thought it would be. It had his characteristic zing, which was nice, but more importantly it was interesting. His paragraph on his selection process for being this year's Sun Run poster boy was a good example of what I found interesting about his stuff. He delved into the real-world motivations behind an editor's facade, then latched hard onto the unspoken insult of the editor's question of whether he wanted to get into shape. It was this depth and vision that I found engaging. But could he run? This was what I asked myself as I reviewed the article.

In the column McMartin mentioned that he lived in Tsawwassen. I had forgotten about that. He wrote about where he lived the year earlier in a biting column that could be subtitled "Yummy Mummies of Tsawwassen." I promised myself at that moment to dive into the recycling heap and reread the first Jenny Lee article of that year's Sun Run to see if there was any indication of which areas of Greater Vancouver Erin Davis and Gwen were from.

You see, Tsawwassen is a community within the municipality of Delta. I already knew Steve Darling was from Delta, and of course I live in Delta. I had no idea where Jenny Lee was from, but I remember thinking that if it should turn out to be Delta, well, I would need to take a page from Poh-Poh and take heed of the mystical and supernatural forces at work. After reading and attributing more signs leading to

Delta in the *Vancouver Sun* than on Highway 99, I'd have had no qualms about quitting on the spot. I'm not big on coincidences being explained away by laws of probability. The math folks in the world would say, "Dave, when it comes to math, your mind is limited, man." They would be right, so I go with what I know. Let there be no question about it, I know what spooks me, and if it had turned out that everybody from Nancy to Jenny Lee was from Delta, I would have just walked away—well, limped on that day—and let the whole running initiative fade to black.

By the time I finished reviewing Pete McMartin's goals, which of course included a fashion-oriented goal of enough weight loss to accommodate some spiffy apparel that had been sitting in his closet for five years, I had completed the training session and found myself at the back door. Overtime, oh yes, he mentioned that he wanted overtime as well for all his training. Didn't I tell you the man was a card? It wasn't until I had closed the door, guzzled a glass of water I had left out on the counter, stretched my calves on the pile of wood, and took a shower that I stopped the stopwatch. I then grabbed the Document off the fridge and sat at the kitchen table to reflect on the last one hundred minutes and record my thoughts on the lines I had previously drawn next to each training session.

First off, I have to tell you that I then felt my breasts. This entirely bawdy and self-absorbed behaviour was all Pete McMartin's fault. He had written about his largeness, and it was my best guess after getting a good grasp of the situation that I probably wasn't that far behind him. My only problem with the breasts at this point arose when walking downstairs, which was very disconcerting because I found the heaving breasts distracting. The corrective action of holding onto the handrail at all times was implemented after a mindless and asinine attempt to gawk at myself on the stairs using the Linda Blair swizzle-head manoeuvre, causing me to stumble and nearly take the type of tumble that results in a full-body cast. The manoeuvre and the movie from which it is derived have been outright banned from the household by Shelly ever since.

After determining that I was close but thankfully not ready for a sports bra, the next body part that I felt was my shins. They felt bruised on the inside edges. I surmised that this was the initial stage of shin splints. Although I'd never had them before, I'd overheard so many people complaining about them over the years that the pain felt recognizable and familiar in a way that was fascinating. I rubbed them a bit then got up, cursing myself for taking the long route with its hard surface to the park last week. I got that bit of concrete running knowledge by eating a hot dog while standing next to a couple of square-jawed guys in suits at an Orange Julius in Pacific Centre shopping mall. Between slurps of what was probably a super-low-fat vitamin-infused banana smoothie, blue suit complained to brown suit that he'd beaten the crap out of his shins on the weekend while running on the street. No, I didn't ask him to show me.

I did a slovenly slide in my socked feet along the cork floor to the pile of wood in the corner of the kitchen, where I stretched my calves out one last time. My shins were sore, but I had run for one minute for nine repetitions, something that seemed like a distant possibility last week, when between running for thirty seconds and contemplating surgery I had spent a great deal of time considering either my shortened life or my imminent death.

After stretching, I was standing there feeling pretty good about myself and thinking that my heel wasn't getting any worse when hunger pangs took full control over all thought processes. I'll never forget seeing a small shake in my hand just before it grabbed the vertical white handle of the fridge door and jolted it open. I then used both hands to frisk each individual shelf for filling foods that were easily identifiable, easy to open, and easy to prepare. My appetite had been reduced over the last week, but on that first day of week two it had returned with a vengeance. I remember thinking during the previous week that with the reduced appetite the weight loss potential was far too high, and it all seemed way too easy. Weight loss wasn't a goal of course, but nevertheless the situation seemed too good to be true, and as it turned out, it was.

The exercise must have traumatized my system, shutting down primary body functions such as the craving mechanism for double desserts. Starting in week two, though, it seemed to spring back to its normal level of decadence. I guess once my system figured out through the pattern of scheduled rest days that dementia hadn't forced a death march on me via Delta's parks, it might as well endure the ordeal on a full stomach. I made up all lost calories that day and probably added an equal number of calories just for good measure. The return of my appetite was leviathan in nature, and according to Shelly so was the mess in the kitchen. It wasn't a pretty site.

Session 2 40 minutes. Run 1 minute, walk 4 minutes. Do this 8 times. Thursday, January 16, 2003.

The next day the doorbell rang, just as I had expected it to. Then it rang again and again, just as I had expected it to. I opened the front door, then leaned partway out of the house as I held open the storm door. I felt a small child brush by, just as I had expected. I then could feel the muscles on the side of my face loosen, and I became slack-jawed. I hadn't expected this. Standing at the bottom of the two-step landing was Nancy, her right arm held high over her head, waving a long goodbye to her daughter, my daughter, and me. She then pivoted on her left foot, revealing for my 180 degree viewing edification a wrist-to-ankle Lycra-sheathed body. I watched the satiny black form on glossy white runners move with great purpose down the driveway, her silken brunette hair swaying in a loose manner behind her.

Nancy was at the end of the driveway before I got out my first *what* inquiry. She raised her hand again, turned her head, and without breaking stride said in her familiar and always cheerful voice, "Thanks." I closed the storm door at the kids' insistence but continued to stare through the glass window at the youthful and vibrant woman as she approached the willow tree. I didn't think she had heard my question, and I had so many more to ask. What kind of shoes were those, what was the price of the Sun Run clinic, what route was she taking, what level was she at? I didn't get even one *what* answered, a truly disappointing performance on my behalf. I watched Nancy, in her new gear and a never-seen-before steadfast stride, pass under the waterfall of willow branches, then I blurted out a *why* that produced a thin fog over the storm window—and she was gone. Why as in what was her motivation?

I closed the sturdy front door, but I couldn't get Nancy off my mind. What was a team leader, how many people were in the clinic, where were they from? I was so taken aback by her image that I had to sit down. Her eyes were bright with enthusiasm, her cheeks rosy red, and she had a vigour in her step that evoked confidence, but most of all the Lycra sheathing shaped her presence into an image that said *power*. Oh, I was slack-jawed all right, but you would be too if the young mum down the street had just turned into a powerbabe and looked as if she could physically dominate you.

I took the kids to the Sungod Pool for swimming that day after Nancy left. I was kind of hoping (well, really hoping) that I would see the Sun Run clinic in action, but they were nowhere to be seen. As curious as I was and as much as the kids liked swimming, this wasn't the reason we had gone to the pool. Like my appetite, which had returned with such gusto, I could feel my energy level coming on strong as well. I could have run on that day of rest no problem. In fact I had a burning desire to, especially after my encounter with the neighbourhood powerbabe, but the training Document said, "Resist the temptation. . . ."

The problem with temptations is, well, umm, let's just say I end up quitting all my temptations, so early resistance was vital if I wanted to meet my goal of attaining fitness by completing the Sun Run program, which included running in the Sun Run 2003. Besides, the training tips section of the Document said I'd just increase my risk of injury. I had enough problems already that had resulted in undue pain, trauma, and anguish, and I didn't need to willfully stack the pile in yet another ill-conceived attempt at measuring (for future reference only) the threshold of my ability to endure excruciating prisoner-of-war-type torture. So I went to the pool instead to burn off all the excess energy.

I guess you could call this either not being fully prepared for being a prisoner of war or just cross-training. I prefer to call it the no-sweat way to have fun since I'm not really an athlete, which cross-training would imply. Plus my POW torture-preparation days were dropped a long time ago under the sternest of advisements by a man whose dispensing fee was paid in the currency of Canadian Tire money.

The next day my apprehension about the Sun Run program was so high that I really could say I was full of fear. It was all because of Nancy, with her confident waves and spins and all. Then her intrepid march towards the Sungod Recreation Centre had been just too much.

Now you may think I was intimidated, but really that wasn't the whole story. A little bit (well, probably a lot), but not the whole story. My next biggest problem was that I was unprepared for the neighbourhood throwing down of the gauntlet. When it comes to me, these things don't need to be written down or verbally tossed about, or as in this case, there doesn't need to be intent. At least I hope this was the case, since Nancy had no idea I was training for the Sun Run. Of course I realized at the time that I was probably hallucinating this whole gauntlet aspect, but it didn't really matter since what really mattered was that I had shaken myself to the core regardless. To add insult to all this, the emotional flailing wasn't part of the plan, and nowhere did the beloved Document say how to deal with this sort of thing.

I lay on the hallway floor thinking about Nancy and doing an unprecedented fourth set of warm-up exercises as I prepared for that day's training session. All this self-imposed stress created a feeling of doing the exercises in slow motion. I've always heard that exercise reduces stress, but my body didn't seem to be responding to this maxim. In fact, I was beginning to think that exercising under such tension might not even be considered a tonic at all when the little dog jumped off the wingback chair in the living room and curled up beside my prone body. Maybe I had been down too long and she sensed an opportunity to sneak in a little companionship time, or maybe she just needed to see what my biggest problem was.

I was giving Rosie a good back scratch when it occurred to me that my response to the throwing down of the gauntlet would be to do exactly what I had been doing all along: concentrating on the basics and staying within my physical limits. I had confidence that good things would happen if I did this and of course stuck to the letter of the Document. Upon concluding my course of action, which really was to do nothing differently, I performed a mental checklist of the warm-up exercises I had completed: sit-ups, knee bends, leg lifts, hamstring stretches, groin stretches, and calf stretches on the painted pile of wood. I would finish off the session with a set of push-ups to drive the adrenalin up and propel me down the driveway.

Before I did the push-ups, I lay there a bit longer, giving extra attention to the little dog. She certainly was sweet and she sure provided me with comfort, but what was her real motivation for circling in on a perfect scratch location? At first I thought that maybe some long-dormant Saint Bernard–style genes had been awakened, then I thought maybe her skin irritation had returned, which garnered a lighter, faster, less-abrasive scratch. It was possible, though, that she was just taking advantage of the chance for an old-fashioned scratching.

Between me, Nancy, and now even the little dog, figuring out this motivation stuff was muddling my mind, so I stored it all in my overflowing cache of conundrums, which I now titled "If Men Are from Mars and Women Are from Venus, Then Dogs Must Be from Pluto." Whatever her motivation, Rosie turned out to be much more soothing than any of the warm-up stuff.

I rolled over and did my grunt-inducing push-ups, then used the moulding from the bathroom door frame in a titanic struggle to pull myself up, hand over hand, to the vertical position. I zipped my denim lawnmower jacket, wound the stopwatch strap around my left fist, and exited through the back door. Seconds later I was fumbling with the keys and the watch as I gained entry through the front door. It was pouring rain, and I could feel the splattering of every cold drop on my sparsely populated scalp because I wasn't wearing a hat.

For reasons that are completely beyond my comprehension, after donning my lawnmower hat I checked myself out in the bathroom mirror. My first reaction was *très bien*, but I may have stood gawking one millisecond too long. The realization took hold that I wouldn't be getting any style awards with all this baggy denim and grey cotton, dappled with dark, wet blotches from the rain. This brought about the fastest light flick-off seen for at least that week.

The one-minute run brought me to the back fence of Audrey and Ted's house. This was good, or at least it was as expected, and next week I would be able to run completely past their house. Oh, I thanked the heavens over and over again that Audrey and Ted weren't standing out on their new deck having a beer and waving at me as I ingloriously walked by.

Once I made it to the Sungod Track, it was time to start running again, and I could feel the pain in my shins. I may have been slow before, but my pace was now downright turtle-like. There was no discernable speed change when the next walking portion came due. On that day the only difference between walking and running was that the running portion had much more of an audio component and much more body bobble. I gritted out the forty-minute training session mostly at the Sungod Track, the exception being the travel time to and from the park. When I got home I made a note on the Document that both shins were now painful, but the heel was a bit better. I just couldn't imagine finishing the training session if I didn't have the soft bark mulch of the Sungod Track to run on.

This day had also been my first in an all-out rain, which strangely I benefited from because the track soaked it up and then had a bit more cushion to it. There had been a mist or light drizzle on some of the previous days—it was, after all, winter in Greater Vancouver. All in all, my run attire worked well in the winter weather. The temperature was just above zero Celsius, so I wore a sweatshirt under the denim jacket. I figured that with so much walking I couldn't get away with wearing only a long-sleeved shirt just yet. The jacket provided loads of mobility, and with its ability to zip up to the neck, it kept the body heat in.

My cotton sweatpants were a brand from a boxing outfit and had an extra-wide elastic at the waist to give them an authentic boxing-ring look. This elastic worked like a girdle, eliminating the need for the enigmatic question of whether the belly goes over or under the belt line; either way it certainly wasn't a Dale Walters bantamweight look. Of course, I also had the baseball hat, which kept the rain off my head, and my glasses. Finally, I wore some dollar-store, lightly woven black wool gloves, which soaked up quite discreetly any of those pesky nose drips.

I was very happy with this ensemble of off-the-closet-shelf stuff. In fact, when I saw a couple of balding running buddies in their fifties, labouring up the steep portion of 112th Street from 72nd Avenue wearing just grey sleeveless sweatshirts, I felt that my contentment was justified. Yes, with their barrel chests, exposed hairy shoulders, and dark circular stains under the pits the world was familiar and in turn a nice safe place. All was fine until I thought of that Nancy and all her National Research Council–tested space-age clothing, then symptoms of a deeper confusion appeared in my life, such as asking Shelly if I looked good wearing this or that and even if I looked fat.

Session 3 40 minutes. Run 1 minute, walk 4 minutes. Do this 8 times. Saturday, January 18, 2003.

Shelly and her shadow, Emma, were both giving me sideways looks as they headed out to do grocery shopping while I lay in the hallway stretching my quadriceps. When the bigger one made an abrupt stop to talk, the littler one bumped into the backside of her cushioned jeans. The Sun Run program was still new in the household, and the two of them were not accustomed to the high level of activity it had brought. Exercising was not the only thing going on. There was a Document on the fridge, alternate daycare pick-ups, showers at odd times of the day, newspaper columns thrown from one end of the table to the other to be read, a new heavy-duty door mat that met with disapproval, and, most of all, talk.

The best thing about all the talk was that I was not necessarily doing the talking. With Nancy participating in the Sun Run training program, both Shelly and Emma would come back from her house full of Sun Run chatter. At this point I was trying to keep my inquiries into all things Nancy as subtle as possible, but as usual I failed miserably at this type of behaviour. I was a touch disappointed in their debriefings after each visit, but it was early in the program and I told them we all had room to improve. Of course that bit of commentary went over like a lead balloon. I was told to go get my own answers, but I knew my interviewing skills left a lot to be desired. So I found myself in a position of having to apologize to both of them and then beg them to continue to be my *what* agents. It always bothers me how much the two of them enjoy the begging. You see, I tend to get myself into these positions often.

When the grocery shoppers closed the back door behind them, the rear windows shuddered, and then, as if on cue, the littlest and furriest one of them all jumped down from her pillowed loft on the wingback chair and assumed the scratch position. Rosie was a fast learner.

I thought I was putting in a lot of stretching time before each training session, but every time I got out on the track, it seemed as if it hadn't been enough. My body felt very much like a pole in its desperate attempt to manoeuvre down the street. An Emily Carr pencil sketch of a totem pole, to be exact. Slightly off-kilter and solitary against a pencilled grey sky, my body (like the totem pole) would be stiff and unbending, and just as a totem pole's assortment of crests and figures depicted trials and tribulations, so too did my various body parts.

Inherent in a totem pole's design is its external decay and internal rot, and I can't say I was feeling much different about myself at this point. I was also on the lookout for which body part represented the Raven—a trickster figure that could be mischievous or even foolish. No part or organ escaped my suspicion. But all in all I truly believed that the base exercising and following the Document to a T would change my current standing as a lousy shame pole into a free-standing totemic sculpture.

With each of my rollovers on the floor, the little dog repositioned herself for optimum attention. Then as I steadied myself for the final set of push-ups, Rosie sauntered away, knowing the end of her having a captive handler was near. Once again, after finishing the push-up set, I used the bathroom door frame to hoist my unwieldy bulk to an upright position. A drop of perspiration trickled into my eye, causing it to sting, and I put a hand up to wipe it as I began to walk away from the exercise zone in the hallway. My right foot, encased in its mesh-panelled baby, landed on an outside edge, and the ankle turned under—fully and completely. My arms flailed about the nearest wall, searching for support but finding only the non-weight-bearing edges and angles of single-point-balanced pictures.

I managed to stay upright by looping and rolling along the wall until I came to the staircase, where I was able to bring the crashing and banging to a halt. I was too terrified to look down. I hopped over to the living room couch and jumped on, with my right foot protruding upward. I dared to take my first look while I was airborne in the flighty hope that if I lost consciousness the landing would revive me. Shock of shocks the ankle was not twisted and bent out of its socket, which of course I found an implausible sight, and once I had landed my mind produced a head-to-toe tremor on par with what I felt the ankle should look like. I propped the ankle up and stared at it in silence. Well, I was silent. My thrashing about had catapulted Rosie into a coughing fit, however.

Minutes accumulated upon minutes, and I was still staring at the offending appendage when the scratching, clanging, and clunking of Shelly's oversized key ring signalled the unlocking of the back door. The collateral damage, from the assault of jagged keys and sharp metal trinkets, would be measured in paint loss. After the hard entry, Shelly stopped and stood under an archway to the living room, her breath short and quick. She carried four bags, two in each hand. There was a sudden release of the groceries, which landed with multiple thuds amid the swishing and crinkling of the plastic bags, the instant she saw my backside positioned flat on the couch.

"So this is part of your new exercise routine?" said Shelly. Her tone was sharp, her enunciation crisp, but her big blue eyes failed in their attempt to produce the Maurice Richard glare. As if knowing this, she turned her back on me and began the process of straightening all the pictures I had knocked askew on the wall. When Shelly touched the first picture, the littlest and furriest one took it as a cue to start wheezing and coughing again. It was ridiculous how just the inkling of starting up the whole whirl of events choked her up. "You know, you are going to be the death of that little dog," said Shelly. She then picked up the bags and stormed out of the room.

You know, it's pretty tough trying to have a conversation when you need to talk over drama dog in the middle of death throes. Anyway, I wasn't able to explain the gravity of my situation let alone garner any sympathy, so I got up. I walked through the living room and into the kitchen, where I stopped and put away the peanut butter on an upper shelf. When I concluded that all lines of verbal communication were down and that my ankle wasn't just some dangling limp lump of its former self, I continued my walk out the back door and down the driveway. I guess this was a big test. I had to prove to Shelly that I was serious about what I was doing. I had to reassure myself that I was committed to keeping to a schedule. And then unfortunately I was back to that prisoner-of-war thing again where I had to push the boundaries of pain and human endurance a bit further.

If in my last training session I had performed in the turtle category, I was now in some even lower station of running, possibly even entering into a caricature of running category. I was so concerned about my right ankle during the one-minute run sessions that I might as well have worn the stopwatch as a monocle. In an attempt to minimize body strain, I decided there was no way I was going to run a millisecond more than one minute, so I became fixated on the display of numbers on the watch from the get-go. Of course, running less than the prescribed time in the Document was not an option.

The right ankle felt tight, with a minimal amount of pain; both shins were still very much factors, but the pain was still manageable; and the left heel still had a bit of the cold dental floss feeling happening. As I listened to the various parts of my body, I thought that individually I wasn't inducing further injury, but when the pain was taken as a whole then coupled with the strain of running up hills—okay, inclines—it left me physically exhausted at the end of the session. It didn't matter that I was running in a sub-turtle category as far as speed was concerned, I was far more exhausted at the end of this session than I was in any of the previous ones. In fact, when I brought the monocle down at the conclusion of the last running repetition and began the final four-minute walk back to the house, I wasn't sure if the fatigue would even permit me to get home. Thank goodness as I wobbled along that there were no soft and cozy snowbanks to drift away in. Needless to say, the final week-two training session didn't conclude with an impeccably timed door opening.

Week 3

Session 1
50 minutes. Run 1 minute and 30 seconds, walk 3 minutes and 30 seconds. Do this 10 times. Monday, January 20, 2003.

I was deep into the intersection of Audrey and Ted's corner lot, with plenty of time left on the stopwatch, when I first saw her. She was more than half my age, as most mothers with buggies are in North Delta, and far too thin to have what sounded like a newborn. She hadn't yet crossed my field of vision from left to right, but by my calculations she would be ahead of me when I came out of the corner—and that was fine by me. After all, she looked as if she was moving at a good clip, and I didn't need the slam-dunk humiliation of being passed by a baby buggy right in front of Audrey and Ted's place. I mean really, who would?

Up to that point it was all systems go as I made a heel check, ankle check, and shin check for my first training session with a run time of ninety seconds. The best part of all, though, was that this would be my first time running completely past Audrey and Ted's place. Mind you, the distance exceeded would be measured by blades of grass on the lawn of the house next door.

I rounded the corner and could see the forest of bare branches enclosing the Sungod Track at the end of the street. I could also see my projected run-to-walk transition point just past Audrey and Ted's. And finally but of the utmost importance I could see that the reed-thin woman pushing the buggy was ahead of me. Then my stomach dropped and I felt a burning sensation rise up and grip my lungs when the young mother bent down on one knee to tie her shoelace. *Get up, get up* I wanted to shout as it became apparent I was going to pass her with far too much time left in the first running repetition. The time left was paramount because it gave her the opportunity to stroll past me.

The woman finished tying her shoe and stood up as I pulled alongside her. This is where, because of my heightened state of terror, I found it oh so easy to blurt out a shameless plea with the woman.

"Please don't pass me."

"Don't worry, you're running," said the woman pushing the baby buggy.

The singsong tone of her reply indicated incredulity at the prospect of being able to pass me, and on top of that she managed to deliver her message with a good dose of morning cheer. Still I didn't trust her—after all, I had seen her speed—so I gave her the same over-the-left-shoulder check that John Landy had given Roger Bannister near the end of their historical sub-four-minute-mile run at the Vancouver-hosted 1954 British Empire Games. Of course, I gave it every couple of seconds just to keep her in her place. The Landy left shoulder check worked better on the woman with the buggy than it originally did on Roger Bannister, because when I transitioned to walking she caught up but did not pass me. The pressure came off as we parted ways at the Sungod Track.

I was later taken by surprise after showering, changing, stopping the stopwatch, and sitting down at the kitchen table to fill out the log portion of the Document when I wrote that my right ankle was fine. It hadn't seemed possible two days earlier when it went under on me. As I reflected on the recent running events, I could only conclude that the reason I was not in an ankle cast was that the sensation I had felt had actually been my ankle slipping in and out of the running shoe. Oh, sure, the ankle bent over pretty good and it was a bit stiff today, but really it was more a case of my mind responding with melodrama.

In trying to figure out some sort of corrective action for my obviously too-loose shoes, I alternated between tying my shoelaces tighter and getting help for the dog. It seemed to me at the time that drama dog was being a bad influence, with all her overreactions and stuff—now I was doing it. Anyway, after adding up the cost of rehab in some countryside obedience school, prescribed veterinary medication, and the time wasted trying to explain, you know, the nuances of it all to Shelly, I took a different direction. Sometimes the easiest solution is the best. So I pushed myself away from the table, tied the mesh-panelled babies a little tighter, and took Rosie for a walk.

Oversimplified corrective action? Not really." Taking the dog for a walk was always good inexpensive therapy for both of us, but on top of that I was hoping for some big-time trickle-down effects. On that day of training I was out there in the elements for fifty minutes, and my perpetual fretting about getting blisters on my feet was only getting worse as the training times gradually increased. So I figured with walking Emma to school and now walking the dog as much as I could, I would toughen my feet up.

Another trickle-down effect of walking the dog was my ongoing effort to have the weather effect on my training be as minuscule as possible. I guess I could have added dog walking to the list of implementation strategies I threw in the garbage back at the beginning of all this. I often wondered if the bravado of the Toller Cranston moment as I tossed out the list was now coming back to haunt me. Could it be that dog walking and how many other brainstormed strategies were similarly tossed and were now not being implemented? Speaking of the beginning, it wasn't too hard to imagine that only weeks earlier I could have put the roof down while driving on a rainy day through a doughnut drive-through and convinced myself that I was truly accomplishing a training objective of weather acclimatization. The times they were a-changing.

Session 2
40 minutes. Run 1 minute and 30 seconds, walk 3 minutes and 30 seconds. Do this 8 times. Wednesday, January 22, 2003.

A very strange thing happened to me during this day of training. Now before you get all worried, let me tell you that I ended up being all right. In fact in the log I wrote that both of my shins and my left heel had been no problem. Then on top of that I wrote, "Easy run, nice and relaxed." Can you believe that? It was as if everything was coming together, but as far-fetched as all that sounds, it was not what made that day's training strange.

I finished my log entry, then pushed the Document to the far side of the kitchen table; in its place I shuffled in this week's Pete McMartin article for rereading. With a practiced hand, I made a small adjustment of the shutters, focusing a narrow beam of dust-free white light onto the article. I was in heavy edit mode as I scrutinized McMartin's words for answers to my dilemma. A smile formed with lightning speed as I reread his opening paragraph, which had a humorous slant in describing one of his running goals. The man wanted to lose enough weight so that he could do his own love scenes. Poor guy, he seemed to have fallen into that borderless and malleable quagmire called weight loss. Anyway, the smile vanished with the same speed as it appeared once I left the text of the opening paragraph. Then in the second paragraph, with absolutely no conscious effort on my behalf, the smile struck again as the man compared his looks to that of a blood sausage. Of course, the smile retreated at the end of the paragraph.

This involuntary facial workout continued for a few paragraphs, but before my cheeks went into spastic shock, I found what I was looking for. McMartin's article that day was on clothing, with most of the ink devoted to his leggings. They were causing him trouble—the fit, the itch, underwear or no underwear. How I ended up with such a fine pair of cotton running pants I guess only Santa knows, but I regress. More importantly, what I found was his description of the type of person who wears this new-fangled athletic clothing.

You see, I had a chance meeting with this type of person out on the Sungod Track that day. I was in the middle of the long backstretch of the looped L-shaped track, headed towards the bottom of the L, when I saw him striding down 112th Street. I had to peer through the barren trees on my left, then across the desolate parking lot and through more trees on the far side of the park, but I saw him all right. His gear was second skin, all black and all tight. Although a sightline existed, there was some distance involved, providing a level of comfort.

Even with my hand out in front of my face, counting down the last remaining seconds of a walking repetition on the stopwatch, I was acutely aware of my surroundings—or at least I thought I was. I know that walking is a means to an end, but that didn't stop me from always looking around to see who could see me walking. It's a bit crazy, but being all geared up and walking felt as fundamentally unnatural as shooting a puck with my wrong hand. The lie of the stick, the angle of the feet, the new elbow hierarchy, the peculiar visual perspective, it all sent out a neural blast of signals saying this is dead wrong.

It was the relative anonymity of the Sungod Track and its surroundings that soothed this savagely twisted and mixed-up emotion that walking created. While its soft, forgiving track was a huge windfall, it was the isolation of the setting that was the driving force behind the slow-motion stepping as I rounded Audrey and Ted's corner lot and got my first glimpse of the track. At least this was how it had been for the last three weeks until that day's training session.

In regimental fashion, I dropped my hand at the final count, then nearly dropped the watch altogether when I found myself facing the man in black. I was surprised that I didn't emit some sort of squeak at the suddenness of it all. The man in black had pro speed, which was good for him as long as he kept it on the street and all, but he didn't. Once the Sungod Pool obstructed my line of sight, he entered the track clockwise to my counter-clockwise direction and was now about to pass me.

He was a tall man whose shapely muscles could be seen flexing with each stride under the gleaming black suit. I didn't notice any Pete McMartin sausage-style body rolls, but I did notice that his most prominent body protrusion was his jutting square jaw, which I fixed my upward stare upon as he neared the point of passing. The jaw began to move, bringing into focus an upper set of sparkling white teeth, and he said, "Good job." And then he was gone. I felt like the victim in some sort of run-by verbal assault.

Good job, what did that mean? Oh, the words lay heavy on me as I sat at the kitchen table, picking up speed the farther I went down McMartin's article looking for a launch point. In his article, McMartin mused about the alphabet of human personalities. I picked what I felt to be the appropriate letter for the man in black, then attained lift off for a review of the Sungod Track incident. I guess I didn't like the fact that the man in black had veered in such an obvious manner off the street before performing some sort of quickie evaluation and pronouncing the sum of his assessment. His lack of tact was an affront to my sensibilities, and frankly, I found the whole thing confrontational. What, he couldn't just hold himself back from checking out the roly-poly rookie?

He not only had a striking physique and a wardrobe that accentuated it, but also, given the fact that he closed down on me within seconds, I could say without reservation that his speed was intimidating. The Sungod Track was supposed to be my sanctuary against the harsh reality of seasoned competitors and the relentless stares of looky-loos. The man in black had single-handedly put that idyllic notion in jeopardy. And once I got over this initial trauma of having my sanctuary stormed—it was a public place after all—I moved on to feeling as if I were some kind of freaky sideshow act. Well, isn't a roly-poly guy tiptoeing through the woods wearing his lawnmower jacket and a stopwatch as a monocle a tad curious? Anyway, after dealing with these truths the review took a turn for the worse.

I tidied up the newspaper, then centred the flower vase on the table, which Shelly had filled with fresh-cut white tulips. I then got a front paw to back paw teeter-totter dance from Rosie when I asked her if she wanted to go for a walk. I needed to get some air to clear my head, and I had to visit the scene of the incident again to help me make sense of it all. You know, despite my quest for privacy, it wasn't as if I was the only one who used the park. The parking lot can be a beehive of activity after three in the afternoon when school is out or on weekends, with children piling out of the passenger seats of a constant stream of vehicles to go either skating or swimming. This particular training session took place during the morning, mid-week, so the activity level was far lower and consisted of adults using the facilities.

Out on the one-kilometre track that forms a closed-loop perimeter for the recreation facilities, Rosie and I met two other walkers (one with a dog, one without) and two runners. The walkers were familiar faces and always gave a smile and a quick "Hello" as we crossed paths, but the runners I had never seen before. Both runners crossed our path swiftly and silently, each giving a small hand gesture of acknowledgement when I said, "Hi."

So far, this cross-section of people I had met represented a typical day on the track as far as behaviour and numbers go. The overall numbers were most likely a bit higher, since the length and configuration of the track meant there could be someone positioned at the opposite end, let's say walking a dog at the same pace, whom I might not ever see let alone cross paths with. Overall the foot traffic was sparse, with the group as a whole considered kind and gentle. The man in black, with his proclivity for an invader-inspired fleet-of-foot modus operandi, just didn't make the cut with this group.

I didn't make it to the exact spot where the incident had taken place because Rosie demanded that we stop at the ice shavings the

Zamboni dumps in small piles at the back of the ice rink. While she made use of the full length of her leash to climb to the top of one pile and nose around, from my vantage point I could see the offending location at the foot of a looming pine tree. In an attempt to understand what bothered me most about the man in black, I took the Poh-Poh angle of it all being some sort of sign, with maybe a metaphor of some type just waiting to be exposed. Or could it be the man in black hit a nerve with his choice of the word *job*?

I mulled this over as Rosie came down from her perch, and we walked until we were under the pine tree and standing next to the first of many homemade footbridges along this section of the track. This one used old railway ties to span a drainage ditch from a residential back fence to the Sungod Track.

Although I had put words to paper every day in true Pierre Berton fashion, my work of fiction (being unpublished and all) was a stretch to being categorized as a job. Besides, not having a nine-to-five place to be every day was how Shelly and I had intentionally set myself up. No, the spoken word *job* hadn't hit a nerve. But the longer I stood beside the gandy-dancer's footbridge, the more I thought that maybe his words hit something else. If not a nerve, then maybe something softer, maybe an innermost feeling, maybe something that touched my heart and soul.

It had taken me a few hours to break through a wall of fierce denial, but yes, I had initially despised everything about the man in black because I enjoyed being told that I was doing a "good job." Hey, I had been at it hard for three weeks now, and I truly am not someone who craves approval from others, but my behavioural change because of running was just so damn strange that it had created an unexpected vacuum of constructive feedback in my life. It had taken me a while to understand the significance of the man in black's comments, but should I ever see him again I would give him a chipper "Hi" and a quick wave, but really I should be saying, "Thanks, I needed that."

I gave serious consideration to the question of my self-esteem on the way home, as Rosie and I stopped only to investigate some unusual dormant bushes that seemed to be renewing themselves by sprouting white popcorn. I revisited my choice of not joining, like my neighbour Nancy, the Sun Run training clinic, where in the camaraderie of pulling together to accomplish a single goal there would be much more of this man in black type of cheerleading. By the time the dog and I got home, I had reassured myself that I had made the right decision and that my motivations to go it alone were healthy, but I guess I just had to be reminded that this business of solo training did have some shortcomings.

Session 3   50 minutes. Run 1 minute and 30 seconds, walk 3 minutes and 30 seconds. Do this 10 times. Friday, January 24, 2003.

The rain in the Greater Vancouver area never ceases to amaze me. I had spent my school years in the prairie city of Winnipeg, where I grew accustomed to a meteorological temperament that fits in on the savage end of the climate scale. In Winnipeg you can be enjoying a fine sunny day, strolling down one of its main streets, which can be as wide as an English Bay freighter is long, and see the impending rainstorm approaching in the form of a single dark menacing cloud. The cloud's trajectory is easy to calculate, in part because of its contrast against a marble-blue sky, but mostly because of its unwavering course. It's possible to dodge this monkey's wedding of a rainstorm by simply crossing the street, with the only concern being whether you have misjudged its speed, forcing you to perform an emergency blast from one side to the next. That single cloud will pass over in minutes, deluging the equivalent of a full day's rain in Vancouver.

It's this dissimilarity that never ceases to amaze me. The Vancouver skyline goes dark from the North Shore mountains to well beyond the U.S.–Canada border, eking out a pitter-patter of rain that throws an envelope of perpetual moisture around you. In Winnipeg you can get a rapid pelting of raindrops that have amalgamated to the size of chestnuts and a good bruising if they turn to hail, whereas in Vancouver it's a long, drawn out case of waterlog, then rot by mildew and mould.

Every once in a while, though, the Vancouver rain cranks it up tenfold to prairie intensity (but without the lightning, thunder, hail, and maiming), as it did on this day's training session. When I looked outside and saw the turbulent flow of the twin rivers in the street gutters, I knew I would have to battle through more than the usual mental constraints and physical shortcomings. Rain at this intensity occurs when the jet stream carries warm, moist air from Hawaii across the Pacific—a route dubbed the Pineapple Express—then dumps it as rain once it reaches Canada's west coast.

At the foot of the driveway, I made a leap across the river, pulled the brim of my hat down to protect my glasses, and was off towards Audrey and Ted's corner lot. It did not take long, just the first walk interval before the Sungod track, before I announced to my inner costume coordinator that I had attained complete clothing saturation. Much to my surprise, I was warm and comfortable. Although I could feel the various layers of cotton pasted to my skin, the outer shell (that trusty lawnmower jacket) remained mostly loose so as not to restrict my movements. I guess through a combination of my body throwing off copious amounts of energy and the cotton jacket smothering most of it, I can say that I wasn't cold. But I sure was concerned.

This was now the end of week three of the training program, but the concern seemed much older than that. I have to tell you, I just did not know if I could go the distance. The time on the track was like an elastic band, expanding and contracting with each session, and it was my luck that on this wet and rotten day the timeline was being stretched out to fifty minutes. Initially my concern was that I would increase my chance of injury the longer I was out there, but on this day of training I just wasn't sure how much weather I could endure.

The track didn't take too kindly to the torrential downpour, either; portions had flooded over where the track ran parallel to the vehicle driveway at the entrance to the recreation facilities. I was forced to share the pavement in these sections. The freshly installed landscaping and the section of track behind the newly constructed Sungod Pool took a severe beating, as it became a mountain of mud. I was forced to yield to an alternate route provided by the construction project planners, which was along the fenceline of the neighbouring properties. The alternate route was flat and puddle free, but why I considered this detour a hardship I believe I will never know, even though I have several theories in the works.

I arrived at the back door of my house with my usual impeccable timing and exhaustion. By the time I had changed, showered, and sat at the table to reflect on the training session, I felt quite a sense of accomplishment because I hadn't let the weather overwhelm me.

I slowly laid my head in my folded arms on the table as I thought of how close and tough a fight it had been—you know, slugging it out in the mud and all—when I spied through my one little eye the Document on the fridge with handwriting all over it. Then I saw the stopwatch, with its strap strewn across the computer station, and a moat of water on the kitchen floor, the lawnmower jacket amassed at its centre. Ah, the regalia of a job well done. But then the single-eye perspective refocused.

I blinked a few times, but my conclusion did not change. I could have made a better copy of the Document after figuring out its role and configuration. I could have made a banner of my mission statement. What was I doing with that stopwatch? It was awkward to hold, and it gave me a headache because of the internal debating that always ensued over what repetition I was on since it didn't have lap-counter capability.

The lawnmower jacket was something else. I can't say if I looked like a dork; I didn't feel like one when I was wearing it, and it sure worked well, but hey, I didn't see anyone else dressed like that, if you know what I mean. No, I couldn't blink the new reality away. These were the vestiges of a lack of permanence. Just how committed was I to this whole running program? I hadn't even put the Sun Run date on the family calendar let alone paid the entry fee. Oh, sure, I guess I was making myself available—you know, for that Sunday family outing for ice cream, followed by a casual stroll to admire the artwork in the park. What was going on here? I needed to start thinking about doing the Sun Run course and running through Stanley Park, not walking through Peace Arch Park.

When it dawned on me that I was leaving the door open so I could close the whole training program down on a moment's notice, it got my dander up. I figured I would raise the quitting stakes and put a little more on the line tomorrow by sprucing things up in the kitchen and purchasing some single-purpose gear. My eye slipped shut at the thought of going retail again.

The next day, I found myself heading towards the uptown business district of Vancouver to get my running gear and feeling mighty fine about it because if all went well, I planned on visiting my favourite stereo store, which was nearby. There was no coincidence in the proximity of the two stores; it was all by design, a lure if you will. But I saw an open parking spot right next to a different sporting goods store, and forces greater than any safe driving incentive took over and had me wheel into the tight spot in expert fashion.

I opened the door, stepped inside the store, then performed a two-handed hair comb—you know, one of my many retail entrances that signal, "Keep the security hounds at bay, I'm clean." Of course, it didn't work, and a sales representative pounced on me. Before he had finished his greeting I had already said, "Running jacket, size large." Holy smokes the guy was efficient: within seconds, he had two jackets in my hand to try.

It was an embarrassment to stand in front of the mirror wearing clothing designed for the physically fit. I tried on both, scared the sales representative away when I laughed aloud after thinking of Pete McMartin's sausage comments, then I too moved on when I saw the price. More than two C notes. I might have cried if I hadn't been laughing at the time. Over at the watch counter was a different sales representative, whom I told I wanted to see watches that had lap-counter capabilities. This seemed to stymie the poor fellow, and I immediately had a confidence breakdown in my ability to convey technical information, or even English for that matter. Was I using the wrong term? Was I mumbling? Or was I just not hip to some new lingo for sports wristwatches? The salesman eventually turned away to select a product for demonstration, and when he turned back far faster than I thought possible, he caught my mouth in the middle of forming the word *counter*. The poor guy, I had him going from eye-opening stymied to eye-opening bewildered in a matter of seconds (believe me, there is a difference; I've seen it). Anyway, at the end of the pitch he gave up the price. Again more than two C notes.

I was beginning to get the big picture of the store when I spotted a familiar low-budget brand of watch in a clear rectangular glass case at the far end of the counter. I asked the salesman about these watches, and he said, "Oh, they don't work." I thanked him for his time, then reprimanded myself as I headed out the door, not only for stopping but also for shopping in the first place.

Minutes later I was parked again and standing outside the stereo store, looking through the window. My anger and frustration were washed away, and before they could be replaced by greed and lust, the sweeping arm movements of the sales staff beckoning me in broke the spell, thank goodness. It wasn't unusual for one of them to come to the door and ask if I wanted to come in for a cup of coffee; sometimes they would even offer to feed my parking meter. The generous, kind folks who work in that store actually care about the interior design elements of my house and seem to have a vested interest in how I would apply their products in my household. The neighbouring businesses are often beneficiaries of their civility, but just the same I realize that their mind control techniques are just a bit more polished than the others, and I rarely go in.

I waved back, then headed up the steep slope of the neighbouring street to the sporting goods store. The first sporting goods store had taxed my patience, insulted my intelligence, and cut my stereo ogling time. By the time I reached the second store, I had ruminated over this poor treatment to the point of being emotionally broken and feared that my ability to complete a shopping transaction was on the verge of becoming nonexistent. So I stopped outside the sporting goods store and looked around for someone to do the shopping for me. I got a few hi's out, but because Shelly worked in the neighbourhood, I was too busy formulating a defence for soliciting women in my version of a mystery shopper to manage anything more than that. So the hi's ended up being just hi's. Fortunately, after going over my defence a few times, the fresh air had cleared my head, and I realized it would be easier to suck it up, suppress my anxiety, step inside, and do the shopping myself.

It was a bright store with an abundance of natural light that illuminated the entire athletic stock. In my steadfast walk to the cashier area, I noticed that I was the only customer in the store. The sales representative had her head down as I continued my approach, and I remember thinking, where had I seen that shade of red hair before? Of course I kept my hands visible by placing them on the glass counter, and that's when she lifted her head to acknowledge my presence.

My torso shuddered and my knees weakened, forcing my palms to press flat onto the glass. It was hideous; dangling from her teeth were bean sprouts, and in her cupped hands, which she held under her chin in an attempt to catch any falling stocks, was the thick, overflowing source itself, the bean sprout, cucumber, and tomato sandwich. Although I was immobilized by revulsion, I was able to get beyond the sprouts by looking her straight in the eye, then said, "Large running jacket, please." The young girl turned her head to the left, then held out her sandwich in both hands, like a sacrifice, to a wall of running jackets.

"Everybody wears those, but they won't keep you dry in rain like yesterday," she said as if she could read my mind.

On the word *they*, the sprouts did a gentle side-to-side sway reminiscent of the neighbourhood willow tree's droopy branches blowing in the winter wind. I diverted my attention from the fresh verdure to the wall of jackets, which I recognized as being a popular choice in the neighbourhood by the cut of the materials in their design, the wide reflective safety strips, and their distinctive colours. When I saw a sign indicating that the price was well under a C note, I said (more to a display carousel than to the salesgirl) that I would take one in red, to which she replied, "Would you like a hat with that?" A loud crunch of the sandwich followed the question, then the young clerk was off. I mumbled a reply after being startled by the last bite, then restated my affirmative answer in a much more emphatic manner when it became apparent that she was moving out of normal conversation range.

I then became absorbed by the watch display on the counter, which looked suspiciously like the display in the previous store, which of course held the watches that didn't work. It didn't take long to choose one; I simply picked the one with the biggest face. When the sales representative returned, the jacket was part of a bundle that she embraced in her skinny, freckled arms then flopped onto the glass counter before me.

When I told her I wanted the biggest watch in the case she said, "You know, your eyesight isn't failing, it's the darkness that's the problem. That's why all our watches have a backlight feature."

I didn't reply to such insight because it smacked of mind control stuff. Instead I investigated how one red jacket could propagate into the bundle of clothing that was before me. A red jacket, a red short-sleeved shirt, a red-long sleeved shirt, a white hat, white socks, and black shorts.

I was peering into the black shorts and seeing nothing but glass countertop when I heard another crunch of the sandwich, causing my neck to tense. I must admit, the tension may have been caused by the fact that the shorts didn't have a lining in them, plus I hadn't really thought about buying shorts. There was no need for them at this point, and besides that, wasn't buying shorts personal? Somehow I felt that Shelly should be with me. I mean, to go with lining or to go without lining, this was the latest shopping challenge I faced as I continued to look at the glass countertop through the second leg opening, figuring that the mesh lining could be stuck all on one side.

"Oh, don't worry about it. Pete McMartin wrote this week that he runs in the kiltish manner. Everything is large except for the shorts. They're extra large."

I could feel my knees going weak again. On top of the watch, the sales representative had placed a key holder, which I picked up and examined for uniformity of stitching. Not only had her mind control techniques probed into the darkest corners of my underwear drawer, she was now privy to my reading habits as well. There was no way I could have looked at her during that moment. It was a losing battle that I wished to end as mercifully as possible, so I nodded in a yes type of way to the key holder, the watch, the clothing, even the McMartin comment, and reached for my wallet. Try everything on, no way. I had to get my extra-large rear end out of there before the hideous yet hypnotic crunching sound had me debilitated to the point where I ended up with new runners.

I never made it back to the stereo store that day; I drove straight home. I'm not sure if it was because of trauma or exhaustion, but either way I knew I was feeling weak-willed and vulnerable to even the most basic mind control techniques deployed at the retail level.

Week 4

Session 1
55 minutes. Run 2 minutes, walk 3 minutes. Do this 11 times. Sunday, January 26, 2003

"Wow, you're going to do all that?" asked Emma. My young daughter was standing behind me, resting her head on my shoulder as I filled out the Document at the kitchen table after that morning's training session. There was a whole lot of information on the Document, along with a whole lot of white space. It was what this white space represented that had captured her imagination on that Sunday just before breakfast. Seventy-five percent of the lines I had drawn next to the newspaper page, which had been pasted to the sheet of typing paper, were blank.

I had no need to look towards week thirteen at the end of the Document to be overwhelmed; I could feel it that very moment as I stared down at week four, session one. It had been a gruelling fifty-five minutes on the track that day, the longest total training time to that point. During the last three walking repetitions, I had found myself giving up wholeheartedly any pretense of walking tall let alone hard. Good posture, form, and intensity were abandoned with the ease of any of the starting dives of the pool's fast-lane swimmers, whom I could see once per lap through the floor-to-ceiling glass windows. I guess what it came down to was either conserve as much energy as

111

possible during the walking portion or place failure to complete a running portion in the highly probable category.

Of course my ability to see the signs of death, destruction, and imminent danger was as finely honed as Poh-Poh's, so I made some adjustments, which included draining my pool of vanity and conceit to unprecedented levels. This had been the first day of wearing my new gear, and getting out there and doing a staggered walk down the backstretch of the Sungod Track should have seemed a decision so perverse as to sicken me, but it hadn't. The winter canopy of bare-branched alder trees down the backstretch had provided more than just protection from the wind, rain, and looky-loos: it had provided the comfortable womb from which the decision was considered.

With Emma chattering away and the aroma of pancakes in the air, I continued to fill out the feedback section of the Document. I had just finished writing that I was surprised my cardio seemed to be further ahead on the conditioning curve than my legs. When Shelly started to set the table for breakfast, I pushed the Document aside. I watched her eyes stay locked on the Document as she worked the table from one end to another; as a result, all the plates and cutlery ended up being slightly off centre at each setting. Oh, she was wary of the Document, all right. I could tell that she sensed it had power far exceeding its humble and haphazard appearance. But she wouldn't talk about it. She didn't even mention anything about my new attire, which I must say I looked just jim-dandy in.

Instead, Shelly started the breakfast conversation by asking Emma for a critique of my reading during that week's Noisy Reading session at her school. I don't know how this got started, but Dad's review had become a regular feature of Noisy Reading. I had received some pretty good scores lately, mostly for good hand movements during page turning. Toller Cranston would have been proud.

"Well, he didn't do too good on Friday, Mom," said Emma.

I could tell that Shelly had stopped eating by the clank of her cutlery on the side of her plate, but hey, I was starving, so I continued the filling process. Besides, most of the reviews started off this way—you know, low technical scores. Shelly always did a few "Oh, sweetie" this and a few "Oh, sweetie" that before she got to the bottom of the problem.

"He wasn't rhyming, Mom," said Emma. What can I say, it was a tough crowd that day. Apparently one little girl's grandmother was far better at rhyming than I was. I told Shelly this was borderline heckling and helped myself to another stack of pancakes, all the while expecting that I would once again be redeemed by the artistic marks. Shelly smoothed things over by telling Emma I wasn't very good at rapping, either. This produced a small smile that allowed them to start their breakfast.

A few minutes passed, and when the second set of marks didn't come in, I went fishing for them. A question here, a question there. My queries were all met with silence, downcast eyes, and a rather large frown (and that was from both of them). I then stopped eating and watched one forkful of Emma's pancakes make a measured journey from plate to mouth, then watched her chew ponderously with unblinking eyes before the words "More timer" emerged laconically from her lips.

I sat back, put my hands in the air, and acknowledged the name of the character from the book I had read aloud. Before I could get a "Yeah, so what's next?" out, Shelly was repeating the words: "More timer." Then she repeated them again and again. Emma's shoulders rose towards her ears in an attempt to muffle the words, which were rapidly approaching the high-decibel range associated with sonic booms. It was beginning to dawn on me that there was a problem when Shelly said, "You're a more timer. The name is Mortimer."

Emma and I looked at each other with expressions as blank as a teacher's chalkboard on a summer day, then we heard Shelly's laughter. It was a jolly jumper laugh that had her hands slapping the wooden table as she bounced around in her chair. Emma turned her head to look at the spectacle to her right, then back to me on her left, and that's when she drew in an enormous amount of air, which produced the loudest and longest series of yuks I've heard in my life. I guess that day's Noisy Reading was the equivalent of flubbing every Lutz and Salchow in a figure skating routine, then tripping on the carpet and knocking over the bench in the kiss and cry area. "More timer" became my moniker for a very long time, but not so much anymore. Once an ignoramus always an ignoramus; I've raised the bar a few times since then.

Session 2 45 minutes. Run 2 minutes, walk 3 minutes. Do this 9 times. Tuesday, January 28, 2003.

Around the year 1827, the North Delta community in the municipality of Delta welcomed its first European settlers, who were attracted by the location on the mouth of the Fraser River and its plentiful supply of salmon. Fishing, canning factories, and berry farms were the staple industries in the nineteenth century. Not much has changed over the years as North Delta continues to be the fastest growing industrial sector in all of Delta.

With the community remaining working class, there are no private palatial residences with sweeping architectural features, like the boulevard to the entranceway of the Sungod Recreation Centre. The boulevard has mature pine trees lining it in a stately manner so that even the most compass-challenged folks know they've reached the park by virtue of its evergreen thoroughfare. I cut across the boulevard and noticed green shoots sprouting at the foot of the pine trees. Ah, winter in British Columbia's lower mainland—the meteorological envy of the rest of Canada every January.

As I walked this bottom portion of the looped L-shaped track, I kept an eye on the Sungod Pool's double-wide automatic doors opening and closing. I found myself doing this the first few laps or so pretty much every training session. All the visible jiggling and jostling of the various parts of my body no doubt continued down deep past the bone and became a waggle and joggle of internal organs. This resulted in a fierce need to go to the bathroom, which of course was just through the pool's doors, making plumbing and hydration facilities two more virtues of training on the Sungod Track.

I had given some thought to reducing my water intake during the warm-up exercise portion of each training session, but in the end I decided that the benefit of having extra water in the system far outweighed needing to go to the bathroom. Besides, I figured my bladder and whatnot had to get in shape as well, or at least they needed to be conditioned to this new physical regime.

Although my left heel was okay, I could still feel some dental floss–type sensation down there, so I continued to stretch daily on the painted pile of wood in the kitchen. The right ankle was also okay, but again I could feel a sensation around it like a rubber band being strained to its utmost limit. The shins were in the same category as well, where they had felt fine for the last week or so yet seemed to be under a great deal of tension, especially at the beginning of each run.

I had an ongoing dialogue with each of these body parts, getting them to report in, pretty much with each tender and softly planted step on the track, which had attained much more cushion recently as its bark mulch became waterlogged in the winter rains. So by the time the internal organ report sloshed in, along with a minor throb in my upper back, I'd had a good accounting of everything for the full forty-five minutes of the training session, and it all left me, well, a little on the jittery side.

Oh, I forgot about the knee report and my underlying deep-seated worry that my extra bulk would blow out some cartilage or pinch off a kneecap. On the dullest days of creativity, I always fell back on imagining both knees going wonky in the same training session. The knee report had not shown any evidence to this point of being worthy of such anxiety-induced scrutiny. Even though at the end of this training session I received check marks in all categories, with all the trend indicators nominally positioned, I still did not feel good about the report. It was as if the trend lines were quivering on the verge of Richter scale explosions one way or another. And those check marks, well, they were shaky individuals; plenty of trepidation had gone into their formation.

All in all, this vast uncertainty that I possessed showed itself in the form of speed, or to be more precise, lack of speed. My comment entry on the Document for this training session read, "Left some in the tank." I could have added *again*, but I was looking at the glass as being half full as opposed to being half empty. In fact at this point in the training, I was looking at this chronic worry as being a real positive. Because if this outlook was saving me from program derailment through injury, then I knew I was going to be successful in this whole Sun Run training thing. After all, I'd been told by various sources—sources with personal knowledge, I should add—that I did the Chicken Little syndrome with the best of them.

By the time I got home the sun had set. Inside, the shutters were closed flat; every light switch had been thrown; Emma and a friend were scrambling, screaming, and laughing; the dog was barking; and the TV news was blaring. Shelly added to the cacophony as she clanged the pots on the pot rack while exhorting a tired, "No running in the kitchen." When it got noisy like that, I often found myself contemplating the household of a friend, who has twins the same age as Emma. So I parked myself in a comfy chair in the living room, beset with a lethal combination of exhaustion and dumfoundedness, my head lolling about as I considered a permanent doubling of the fun. And then the doorbell rang.

It was Nancy, Emma's friend's mother, aka Sungod Sun Run Team Leader. She had come after her latest training session to pick up her daughter. Nancy stood by the front door chatting with Shelly while I observed from the living room. From this angle it looked as if the powerbabe was slimmer from head to foot. I dare say, it looked as if she had lost weight. I remember thinking, *Why haven't I lost any weight?* before I tried to lob in a few long-distance questions from my chair, but like blowing smoke rings, they drifted a senseless trajectory, first one way and then another beyond their ears. If I was going to get any answers about the Sun Run, I needed to lift my ample rear end out of the chair and do it face to face.

Now, I had seen Nancy a few times since Shelly had told me she was going to be a Sun Run Team Leader, but it was only for glimpses that periodically turned into fleeting moments, with the first and only question being "Where do you run?" You see, I was kind of obsessed with this question since it seemed that North Delta was nothing but a community of graded hills. In fact at this point I was considering running the Sun Run entirely on the Sungod Track—it was close to home, I wouldn't have to pay for parking, it wasn't crowded, and so on and so on.

Anyway, like some Bulgarian weightlifter, I placed my palms on each arm of the wingback chair. I then repositioned my hands, made adjustments to the angle of the elbows, and closed my eyes in an attempt to marshal the extraordinary strength needed to lift myself out of the chair's soft hollow. Before I could make any headway, I heard a thud and a whole lot of moaning. I opened my eyes to see Nancy at Shelly's feet, writhing in pain on the hard surface of the cork floor. While Shelly twisted and turned, looking for something to grab on to in an attempt to maintain her own balance, I figured from the positioning of Nancy's hands that she had a hamstring in contraction.

My ascent out of the chair was effortless once it became a damsel-in-distress rescue operation. As I strode across the room, Shelly stumbled backwards out of harm's way into the relative safety of the kitchen. When I reached our fallen neighbour, I proclaimed the ability to help her if she would just give me her ankle. I felt a hand on my shoulder, then heard a husky voice say, "Not so fast, buddy boy." I did a slow turn, half expecting the bulging proboscis of Karl Malden. Much to my relief it was Shelly, who said, "We don't do that move around here anymore." The accompanying nasty scowl and evil stare had me backpedalling to the point of sitting in the chair and watching Nancy massage her leg back into shape while Shelly stood guard against "the move."

Oh, boy, the move. How quickly I forget. A couple of months earlier, pre–Sun Run training, Shelly's hamstring contracted on her, and I performed what I called the football move. You know, before a football game all the players buddy up on the field, with one guy on the ground and the other leaning heavily into an upright leg as they stretch out their hamstrings. Well, the move as translated from B.C. Place Stadium to the Hutchinson household entailed Shelly with one leg up as she lay on the carpet, with me straddling her head while I lassoed the upright leg with a towel, then pulled with considerable might.

All was well until I started drooling. Great, elongated gobs. For the life of me I don't know why this viscous expulsion occurred, but needless to say after the ensuing hysterics and the rearranging of my sleeping accommodations, the football move was banned for all time. So this is what Shelly was guarding against. I could drool *over* the neighbours, but she was adamant that I not drool *on* them.

Session 3   50 minutes. Run 2 minutes, walk 3 minutes. Do this 10 times. Thursday, January 30, 2003.

Of course, Nancy survived the spasmodic flop-out to live and run another day. Lo and behold, two days later when I was changing out of my day clothes and into my running gear, I noticed that like Nancy I too was slimming down. The quantitative data supporting this observation was the fact that I had reclaimed a notch on my belt. I must have moved the clip on the belt back and forth ten times between the position of the day before and the latest position before I accepted the fact that I had lost some weight. I was feeling so over-the-top good about the single notch that when I stepped onto the road I had to give myself a reality check. I pulled up the lightweight red sleeve of my running jacket and checked the digital watch on my wrist. Yes, I had completed the warm-up session, or at least I had put in twenty minutes, but I didn't remember much of it. By the time I got on the Sungod Track, I was feeling even better about myself as I reviewed the new running gear.

All in all, my latest shopping excursion had turned out to be the best shopping experience of my life. First off, everything fit, albeit untucked or unstrapped, but I felt comfortable. The jacket's midsection was stretched to its limit, but it didn't look unseemly. And besides, things were changing in this area—but of course that wasn't a running goal. With its zippers, straps, reflective safety stripes, and pocket pouch with waist strap, the jacket was way too functional, but it only beat out the lawnmower jacket when its short drying time was factored it. This was more a measure of how good the lawnmower jacket was than anything else.

Drying was a determining factor in the shirts as well. The running shirts were pretty much a technical marvel. I had never worn one before and found myself pulling out a magnifying glass to examine it after wearing it the first time. The shirt worked like a machine as it pulled the moisture away from my skin, then converted the moisture to vapour to be done with it. I can envision future shirt machines incorporating a system to measure and monitor the body's hydration.

In addition, the watch was far superior in both fit and function to the stopwatch. It was cheap, and of course it worked just fine. The key holder was ingenious, but the best of everything was the hat. Oh, the hat worked well. It had the same technology as the shirt, where moisture was wicked off the top of the head, but it also let heat out and acted like a one-way check valve in that it didn't let rain in. The hat also had absorbent material in the band, which kept the sweat out of my eyes. Of course it had a brim, which kept the sun out of my eyes, but the brim design was wide enough that it also kept the rain off my glasses.

These materials all washed easily and came close to drying during the spin cycle—real space-age stuff. As an added bonus, the shirt machine-cleaned my glasses like nothing I'd ever tried before. Once I slipped, zipped, tied, and strapped on this remarkable costume—including the mesh-panelled babies—I became a psychological and physiological powerhouse. I was able to run with my head held high, breathing through both my mouth and nose for an incredible two minutes, all at once.

I must have felt good. On my third two-minute run, three-minute walk set, I picked up the pace during the walking portion. I was in a groove. I was strong, I was unwavering, and I had a cast-iron discipline forged from a deep sense of purpose. By the sixth two-minute run, three-minute walk set, there was a steadfastness in my stride, and I felt a sense of order coupled with a clarity of vision that is possible only through the achievement of a predetermined and planned objective. By the eighth set I had complete control and a conqueror's quest to build monuments, but just before religious fervour set in, one of late novelist Carol Shields's characters took hold of my thoughts.

From an apparel point of view, I may have recently taken a page from the man in black's manuscript, but during this training session I found myself aligning with the indomitable spirit of Cuyler Goodwill. The fictional Cuyler was a man of character, a man of principles, values, and absolute sincerity. Cuyler was a man whose commitment took the long-view approach, where he put his resolution to the test, one stone at a time. While Cuyler laid or gathered stones on a daily basis to attain his goal of building a memorial, I had come to understand that I was travelling on a parallel path of equal determination, although I was doing it every second day, one step at a time.

On the tenth and final two-minute run, three-minute walk set, my super-charged emotional state of well-being took over, and I quickened my pace heading down the backstretch of the track. Oh, it felt good, so I went a bit faster. I had changed gears twice and the legs were fine and my breathing hadn't changed, so I switched gears again, then I dug even further for an astonishing fourth speed change. I could hear my feet churning up the bark mulch.

My vision of the canopied backstretch became a tunnel, and in the light at the end of it I could see a dachshund. It was little Ollie, who always stopped puttering around in the yard with his owner to take a look at me as I completed yet another leisurely loop of the track. On this loop, however, I was moving at pretty much an uncontrollable speed, and my thoughts were *Stay out of the way, little one!* Ollie's house is next to a chained-off back-access road to the ice rink, and as the mesh-panelled babies ripped the loose grit on the pavement when I crossed it, the dachshund looked up and gave me a single sharp bark.

I completed the two-minute run shortly after leaving the little dog in my dust. Incredibly, my first thought after I gasped for air was that I could have dug down even further and gone even faster. I was shocked at this thought because my memories of such glorious speed had long faded, and to think that I could go even faster seemed like a breach of some kind of law of nature. Needless to say, the speed obliterated any hope of having an impeccably timed session-ending entrance through the back door.

Week 5

Session 1
60 minutes. Run 2 minutes and 30 seconds, walk 2 minutes and 30 seconds. Do this 12 times. Sunday, February 2, 2003.

A curious thing happened after the last session, when I had Ollie the dachshund in my sights and ended up smoking him. I came down with a bad case of remorse. Oh, no, it had nothing to do with the little dog. I would have leaped in the air to avoid him and skidded chest first, leaving some of my old-growth hair on the access road if it came down to it. No, as I sat on the wingback chair rubbing my sore knobby knee and listening to the depressive-toned ramblings of a young Burton Cummings, I had regrets about the speed.

Let there be no doubt that the feeling of having all pistons firing on high was seductive, but I knew then just as Randy Bachman's guitar brought the recording to a harrowing halt that the speed thing was over. Why? Because as I was experiencing physical pain, I recognized the opening volleys of emotional anguish. I knew with certainty, based on experience, that these were early range-finding emotive strikes. They would become violent streams of thought as I searched my soul for the reason I had succumbed to the need for speed and more importantly stepped outside the boundaries of my Sun Run training mission statement.

I pushed myself up and out of the chair and limped to the CD player. I pressed the open/close button, took out the Guess Who CD, and put it in its jewel case. I pressed the button once again, the transport tray closed with a gentle whir, and the system became mute. I guess the follow-up CD should have been the apocalyptic meanderings of Jim Morrison, but just because the speed thing was over didn't mean I was ready for the end.

I limped onward in the direction of the fridge, and once there I ripped the training Document off the door and threw it—clipped magnet and all—onto the table. Moments later, once I had caught up to the Document, I read the writing in bold red ink along the top. "I am going to attain fitness by completing the Sun Run program, which includes the Sun Run 2003." I then looked at the three arrows coming out of the sentence. The first arrow was from the word *fitness*, with the word *goal* written at the end. The next arrow was from the word *program* and had the word *plan* at the end of the point. The third arrow was from the phrase *Sun Run 2003*, and I had written *timeline* after that arrow. I reread the mission statement again, then I reread the entire training Document. Where oh where was there any reference to the word *speed*?

Of course, there wasn't any great discourse on becoming the next Dirty 30. I just wanted to get it done, you know, safely. I didn't need to have a flashy nickname like Jim Young, the B.C. Lions wide receiver from the seventies who had blazing straightaway speed. I didn't want to emulate those electrifying fly patterns of yesteryear. I didn't want the attention of devoted fans let alone their hysterical and impassioned screams of encouragement. I wasn't out to create records or smash personal-best times; in fact, I didn't even have a PB to chase. No, I just wanted to attain a modicum of fitness and complete the Sun Run without pain being part of the equation.

I pushed the Document away and adjusted a shutter angle slightly so that I could get a better view of a puddle in the street that was being pounded relentlessly by the winter rain. *Where did I go wrong?*

was the domineering thought until I couldn't take it any more, and in a desperate need for comfort I picked up a fat medium-point blue pen. I then lunged and snagged a section of the newspaper from the far end of the table and wrote the phrase "Direct cause" in the white space of the newspaper header. The snug sensation of the pen's point moving atop the soft padded pages brought instant relief. Witnessing the wet and inky blue scrawl as it contrasted against the black ink of the newspaper was just the icing on the cake. *Speed* with an overgrown capital S was of course the next word written. I then found a bigger piece of white space and, legible to my eyes only, scribbled the phrase "Contributing factors."

This writing on newsprint was one part of the three Rs of newspaper reading that I picked up from my dad, who passed away many years ago in the early nineties. Reading of course was the first R, ripping was the second (as in ripping out articles), and then writing was the third R as his pen met the freshly torn print and made an annotation. These articles would then sit atop my bachelor father's gummed and grimy ornate Victorian-style coffee table or in a drawer of the matching telephone table, to be pulled out at a later time for either consideration or conversation.

For the life of me I couldn't help but touch a large protruding and calcified bump just below my right kneecap after I wrote down *bursitis*. I got up, made a cup of coffee, and thought about how this ancient football injury (next to today's weight issue) was near the top as far as reasons for taking it slow. By the time I sat down with my coffee, I had ruled out moving "renewed bursae sac inflammation" to the root cause category. The pain seemed to emanate from the side of the knee, not the front, but I couldn't rule it out as a contributing factor.

Next up as a contributing factor was the ankle twist, which was then given consideration for being the root cause. Who would have thought that years of inactivity and father time would collude to rob me of the essential coordination to pick my roundness off the floor? Although the right ankle was still a bit stiff fourteen days later and I was probably unconsciously compensating my running stride somewhat, I eventually decided that it wasn't serious enough to move to the root cause category.

Next I wrote down something I had been suspicious of for the last week or so: quad stretching. After four weeks of diligently following the program, I had not changed my initial heavy-duty, full-course, adrenalin-spiking pre-run exercise routine. I had been thinking of cutting back on this pump-up-the-jam technique, so to speak, and the quad stretching was first on the chopping block. It had found its way to the chopping block because I thought I was doing more harm to my knees than good to my thighs. Not that I felt any pain in doing the exercise, but with my predilection for looking out for my knees, the exercise just felt uncomfortable, even unnatural. The quad stretches weren't the root cause, but they stayed as a suspicious activity in the contributing factor category.

The blue ink weaved in and out of stylized fonts, then whipped around the peripheral edges of photographs and raced along thick borderlines as I contemplated the fundamental reason for injuring my knee. I remember stopping the pen but not lifting it from the newsprint and fixing my eyes on the expanding inkblot. I swirled left, then right, attempting to escape the unavoidable conclusion that was materializing, which if corrected would prevent further knee problems and most likely enable me to complete my training. The root cause of my speed problem was weight loss. It seemed that my recent belt notch movement had caused me unexpected and unaccustomed euphoria, which was directly responsible for my acting out of character.

Well, I didn't need to put much more thought into that. I glossed over the corrective action aspect of my knee injury and immediately jumped to implementation mode as I got up and made myself a cheese sandwich. I had enthusiastically formed the delusion that all would end well if I returned to my conservative nature and reinstated a speed restriction. I would do this by giving new prominence to my obsession with the Document and of course by addressing, with my jaw jutting forward and in the open position, my compulsion for overfeeding. At the time I thought the choice was easy. Either fail in some rapid yet ecstatic manner and view a scalpel from a supine and torturous angle in someone else's hand or maintain the slow and gluttonous convention of the day and win while clutching cutlery over my head.

I was back on the Sungod Track on the third day after the burst of speed session. This had been the first three-day break since I had experienced that dental floss feeling in my left heel after day one of the Sun Run program. Since I'd placed full trust in the Document to see me through to the finish line at the Sun Run, I figured this was the longest break I could take before the Document's published weekly timeline began to be interfered with. Running on back-to-back days or even missing a scheduled training session became possibilities if you started dipping into the fourth day off. I didn't want to be in the position of considering either of those two possibilities, so I stayed on top of the task by keeping my foot on the throttle, so to speak.

Now, I may have had my foot on the throttle, but as I made my way along the track I wasn't exactly twisting the ball of my toe against the trail or the metaphorical floorboards; in fact, it was just the opposite. I found myself trudging along in the most exhausting of manners. A combination of a wet, heavy track burdening the mesh-panelled babies; the extra day's rest sucking the wind out of me; and the mental fatigue of assessing each weight-bearing step on my right knee made this training session overly long and rather uncomfortable.

On the cool-down walk home, Nancy stopped her truck as she drove by, and we talked training. Once again I had trouble getting out any questions beyond "Where do you run?" You see, I still had a morbid fear of North Delta's gradual grades based on my initial road-running experience. The biggest reason I didn't get off many questions, though, was Nancy. She had me under interrogation and showed no compunction whatsoever as she fired off her own laundry list of inquiries. Nancy ended the conversation with a sharp click of the truck's manual transmission dropping into first gear and passed

along one final comment: "I'll bring them by tonight just after six."
She then let the clutch out and zoomed down the street, her long hair
flapping out the open window. I wasn't expecting that, *them* being the
Sungod Sun Run training clinic. Oh, what great fun.

Session 2 50 minutes. Run 2 minutes and 30 seconds, walk 2 minutes and 30 seconds. Do this 10 times. Tuesday, February 4, 2003.

For the second session of week five I was back on the track, back on the every-other-day schedule, and back to being slow. Although it was not raining, pools of water had collected on the trail, forcing my head down for navigational purposes and creating a zigzag line of running/ walking. The water avoidance tack made me feel as if I was staggering, and when this was coupled with the chest pains I was experiencing, it made this the worst training session ever. Oh, I didn't think I was having a heart attack or anything of the sort. I knew at the time what was going on: I was suffering from the adverse effects of change.

It seemed the extra time I had gained from making a change to my pre-run exercise routine had been reallocated to, I guess I could say unsafe work practices, or maybe just say that I was losing focus . . . again. I had removed twenty-five minutes from my set-up time by eliminating the sit-ups, push-ups, knee bends, and adrenalin-producing stair climbing. Good riddance to the sit-ups; all they did was induce body noises that have yet to be properly catalogued. The push-ups were somewhat interesting because the hundred I was doing over three sets during the last month had started to show some real he-man results. However, becoming Charles Atlas wasn't part of the plan. Plus the sit-ups produced a body tremor and a lingering pain in my upper back that I'm sure were both due to this overexertion. Quad stretching and the resulting knee bends wouldn't be missed either, if only to reduce my Poh-Poh–like fatalistic tendencies.

The capper to my pre-run exercise program had been a single burst up the stairs to the second floor. I would walk slowly down the stairs and out the door, down the two-step landing, then slowly down the gentle slope of the driveway before starting to run once I hit the roadway. You know, it was like getting some momentum behind you, but the fact of the matter was I didn't need that anymore. At this point in the training, I was good to go almost from the moment I slipped the mesh-panelled babies on. When I eliminated the stairs I felt it was my biggest achievement to date since it indicated that my participation in the Sun Run training program had gone beyond the need for Herculean effort and was now in the familiar realm of struggling with considerable apprehension. The new bottom line was not so much *if* I could do it but *would I be able to* do it? Anyway, it meant that change had taken place.

Again, based on the experience of an older guy assessing the effects of change in his environment over many years, I should have known better. The change in this case was a considerable twenty-five-minute reduction in the overall training session. The resulting benefit of reduced training time fulfilled an implementation strategy, which I felt I needed in order to complete the Sun Run. I believed that if I could configure my training session slowly over time to be as short as possible, it would increase my chances of being successful. This was all fine if you believe that making change is a neat and tidy linear event. Well, that's never been my experience, and in this case the inevitable chaos emerged, with the result being heartburn.

I should have seen it coming. All I did was fill the newly acquired block of time by filling my stomach. It wasn't a three-course meal with a final gorging on some Eaton's Red Velvet cake; no, it was just a scone. Nevertheless, I was feeling it big time as I belched along a flat portion of the track. Thank goodness for the walking portion, with its time allotment of 50 percent during week five. I needed every second.

Up to this point I had always run on an empty stomach, usually in the morning. If I ran in the afternoon it was usually three hours or so after eating. Who would have thought that twenty-five minutes could result in such a mindless act? I guess it could have been that, just a mindless act, or it could have been a sign that overconfidence was setting in. Whatever the case, I promised myself I would never eat before running again.

By the time I noticed the bitter coldness on my feet, it was far too late for an effective remedy. The sharp pain in my chest, the nausea, and the consequential eye squinting had turned my zigzag circumnavigation of the puddles into staggered lines along the track, with a complete disregard for the accumulated water. I was essentially running along the trail by feel, using the soft and squishy grassed edges as my tactile cue to either cut left or cut right. With failure imminent (that is, not being able to complete a scheduled Sun Run training session—an unprecedented act), I reached back in my memory bank for a positive mental image to help me get through the run, wet feet and all.

What I found was the Sungod Sun Run training clinic running past my house. This brought an instant smile to my face as I recalled the shocked tone in Shelly's question, "Is that your car?"

"Yes, yes. Quick, turn out the lights and sit beside Emma."

"Why are you parked backwards? Why are your lights on? Is it running?" asked Shelly as she stood with a finger on the final light switch.

I finished swinging the kitchen shutters out of the way and sat beside Emma, who had Rosie in her arms. "No, it's not running. Quick, turn off the light."

"What are we looking for?" asked Emma as she looked out the window, now unencumbered by any coverings.

"David, why are we sitting in the dark with spotlights pointed at the neighbour's house?" Despite Shelly's vocal objections, I noticed that she had nestled her chair in close to the optimum viewing area so as not to miss anything.

"That's why," I replied as I pointed across the darkened kitchen table and down the twin beams of light that penetrated the winter's night. "Nancy is bringing her team by."

We sat in silence as the outline of two tall figures identified only by the length of their reflective safety strips exited the blackness on our right, ran through the car's illumination, then faded into the night on our left in a matter of seconds.

They were followed by another group of two, then a group of four. A group of five or six loped by, then back to a group of two. The Sun Run training clinic runners were dashing by in dribs and drabs. Upright torsos and turned heads as they talked to each other defined their features. But because the movement and the intensity of the reflective strips on the running outerwear held me in a trance-like fascination, I could not determine their genders let alone single out Nancy. A group of just over ten emerged, running three or four abreast, which broke the silence in the kitchen as oohs and aahs began to slip from the Hutchinson family. The grand finale was a tightly contained thirty-member swarm of excited energy strips jostling by for our viewing pleasure. All in all, it was a triumphant display of human achievement.

"That was cool, Daddy," said Emma as Rosie wiggled in her lovingly crossed arms, sensing that the big show was over.

"I think suburbia is finally getting to you, Hutch. We'd better make plans to launch the SUV to Salt Water City and see the fireworks this year," said Shelly.

I made it through that training session vowing to never eat before running again and once again thankful for the safe confines of the Sungod Track, which kept the vehicles and other pedestrian dangers out of my way while the mental projector burned brightly throughout the training session.

Session 3 50 minutes. Run 2 minutes and 30 seconds, walk 2 minutes and 30 seconds. Do this 10 times. Thursday, February 6, 2003.

During the next training session I continued with the Cuyler Goodwill approach of taking one dogged and determined step at a time, or as in his case, one stone at a time. While Cuyler was building a monument to lost love in novelist Carol Shields's Governor General's Literary Award–winning book *The Stone Diaries*, I was building a Goodwill Tower myself, but of self-doubt and insecurities. You see, this was my last training session of officially walking. The tipping point in the training Document would come in the next session, where I had to run more than I walked. I wasn't looking forward to that because I simply did not know if I could do it.

Oh, it wasn't the knee or at least the knee alone. The inside edge of the right knee wasn't exactly sore, but it did feel swollen. For the two days between sessions I had been finger probing it with alarming frequency as I checked on the swelling, but it wasn't really swollen, it just felt that way. This conundrum only added to my wariness of breaking through the run/walk threshold. The unavoidable training Document moment of having to come to terms with being a runner was bearing down on me during this session, and no amount of escaping into a famous British Columbia novelist's character was going to lessen the inexorable anguish that was enveloping me.

On the final lap of the session, I trudged up the muddy incline on the backside of the newly constructed swimming pool, then placed my hands on my knees and hung my head until I had recovered enough to walk a straight line home. I had no recent experiences of running in adulthood with which to comfort my mind; I was bone tired from spending the last five weeks getting myself to this run/walk point; I had gone shopping—more than once; I had overcome injuries, and in fact I was injured again. Not knowing if I could run had become too much and had left me exhausted on my feet, so once I got through the back door I walked past the turning point for the shower and headed straight for the couch and lay down. I closed my eyes, then heard Rosie's nails scrambling like mad on the smooth kitchen floor at the unexpected site of me on the couch (at this time of day, I should add). The reckless thumpity thump thump continued across the carpet before I felt her harsh landing on my chest.

I awoke to my wife's pronouncement of "Dinner's ready." Oh, boy. The first thing I did was look at my watch. It said that my last lap was five hours and fourteen minutes long. Wow, going comatose after a training session had never happened before, and I cautiously sat at the kitchen table and attempted to gauge the atmosphere in the household before eating.

Shelly sat in silence, which of course meant the littler one sat in silence as well. They had me cornered with a plate of steaming mashed potatoes, placed in a tactical manner under my nose. I refused to either dig in or ask how I had offended them this time. That seemed pretty obvious since I hadn't picked Emma up from that day's after-school care, plus I wasn't totally awake at that point. Thankfully, Emma broke the silence first as I pondered using my tongue as a utensil while staring into the soft, creamy top of the mashed potatoes.

"So, are you still wearing those dirty runners?" asked Emma.

I leaped from the table, charged into the hallway, kicked off the mesh-panelled babies, flew back to the table, picked up a fork, and had a scoop of much-needed nourishment in my mouth before I sat down. Oh, it felt good. After all, I had missed a meal with that extended nap.

We all ate in silence, while I admonished myself for entering an unlit hallway so readily while Shelly had that "mean ma" look about her. There should be a law against appropriating beauty for such purposes. It took until dessert before Shelly opened up with "You were talking in your sleep again. Have another Miles Davis dream?" The layer of dried salt on my skin forced an uncomfortable scratch, then I felt a head-to-toe chill. I didn't really want to get into that, especially with Emma sitting there with pursed lips and all waiting for a reply, as if she knew what her mother was talking about.

You see, Shelly thinks that Miles Davis recordings are murder music, and although they haven't been banned (like "the football move" or even the movie *The Exorcist*), I don't play any of MD's Plugged Nickel sessions or earlier stuff in her presence. So anyway, Shelly uses Miles Davis as a euphemism for anything to do with crime-fiction, whether it be on TV, in books, or in your dreams. I gave a shrug, spun the dessert plate for a better eating angle, then thought that since I was being served my favourite—pumpkin pie—I was probably reading all the negative body language on display incorrectly, which of course wouldn't have been the first time.

Confused and not knowing what was coming next, I reluctantly whispered, "Not really," while hoping beyond all hope that this would somehow lead to a second piece of pie.

"Well, who is Bird, then?" asked Shelly, which was quickly followed up with a "Yeah" from her shadow.

I quickly surmised that Bird was Charlie Parker, a Miles Davis bandmate who went by this moniker, and that my wife was coming at me from a wicked, improbable, yet highly inventive angle. I began to consider whether a second piece of pie was worth delving into this uncharted territory when it struck me that, for the third time in as many minutes, I had it all figured out wrong.

"What did I say?"

"Gotta talk to Bird, gotta talk to Bird. Over and over again," said Shelly.

I put my fork down, placed both elbows on the table, and assumed a confessional profile by looking away from the two of them out onto the street. I remember thinking I would sound like a madman, but only because they didn't know how the loneliness of being out there on the track brings about delirium. Not that it's a bad thing, but it's usually a private thing. But then again, maybe an old-fashioned state of delirium explained the dinner table husband–wife communication misinterpretations. Besides, I felt obliged to tell them something since they still seemed upset with me, and I felt that if didn't cough up something soon the fate of the pie would be sealed.

"Denny Boyd," I said.

Shelly pushed her plate away and repeated the name with the incredulity of a southern California prosecutor who had just heard the O.J. Simpson not guilty verdict; Emma's lips just got thinner and tighter. "I know him. Why do you gotta talk to Denny Boyd?" asked Shelly.

I was first introduced to Denny Boyd back in 1982 during his second stint in the *Vancouver Sun* newsroom. Of course I had never actually met Denny Boyd, and neither had Shelly. We found him long before we found each other and got to know him and his honest approach, as many other readers had during the course of his thirty-some years as a *Vancouver Sun* columnist.

Denny Boyd the "legula" (a co-worker expression of endearment between Archie McDonald and Denny Boyd) guys home turf for many years was the bottom of page three, five days a week, where he was best known for his articles on the human condition. A typical Boyd column would be his take on a personality such as Thomas Scallen, the American businessman responsible for getting Vancouver its National Hockey League franchise but who years later was shunned by the city and everyone involved in the game. Boyd's column evoked an unexpected consideration for the social pariah, with writing that showcased his ability to detail with fine distinction the man's existence. It was typical Boyd, stuff readers of the *Vancouver Sun* had grown accustomed to.

But getting back to my introduction, the date was March 29, 1982, when my father introduced me to Boyd and the greatest opening line I have ever read in the *Vancouver Sun*. I was living with Dad at the time, having moved out from the windy city of Winnipeg a few weeks earlier. Mum and Dad divorced in 1967, with Dad eventually ending up in Vancouver while Mum raised my sister Meghan and me in Winnipeg. As I wrote a letter home at his kitchen table, which faced a plethora of tall cement buildings in Vancouver's West End, I heard the ripping of a newspaper. The ripping was long. In fact, it was done in such a protracted and slovenly manner that I had to call upon only languorous head-turning speed to catch the melodramatic end of the big rip.

There was Dad, sitting in his threadbare and unbuttoned pajamas on the end of the couch. From my seat across the room, I could see a trembling in his hand. "Boy, have you read Denny Boyd today?"

It was a rhetorical question, which of course I did not answer, but I kept my eyes fixed on him and saw his emaciated body shake as he began to lift himself. He rose before the strewn newspaper on the Victorian-style coffee table, one hand clutching the torn newsprint and the other a fistful of blue-striped cotton fabric of his pajama bottoms, which he wore about where one would strap a saddle on a horse. His unbuttoned pajama top exposed a chest that protruded rather unnaturally in its centre, forming a sharp up–down Rocky Mountain ridge, with smooth glistening lines of scarring running first parallel to it then perpendicular. It was the sticks-and-stitches sight of a man recovering from open-heart surgery.

The shuffle across the room for the hand delivery of the Boyd column took so long I'm sure yellowing of the newsprint had set in, but with the lighting effects in Dad's place I would never know. You see, he had this ugly orange shag carpet that tainted everything with a strange and peculiar glow; colour was rendered truthless.

I remember wearing shorts because the thermostat was set high, and I had to peel myself off the vinyl covering of the kitchen chair for the hand-off. I put out my hand, but when Dad realized he would have to cross his arm across his body, he just dropped the column and continued his shuffle towards the stove to make himself another cup of instant coffee.

I saw the picture of Boyd wearing a checkered sports coat staring up at me as I bent over to pick up his column. The high pile of the shag carpet allowed me to easily position my fingers under the paper, affording me the opportunity to turn it and read the all-capitalized opening line on the way back up. "I AM NOT A MORAL DEGENERATE." Delving headfirst into the line like that stunned me and forced me to retreat back to the column's caption of "Alcoholism: A demon destined to kill" and consider the context of the sentence. But before I could venture into the second sentence, Dad's pajama bottoms caught my attention as he stood before the stove pouring boiling water out of a small cooking pot into his cup. (This was not a kettle or teapot habitat.) The pajamas had fallen down his skinny legs like a hoop over the shrunken staves of a whisky barrel. You know, it's not as if I didn't know—I did have a lifetime of supporting knowledge—but the silent and still image confirmed that, unlike whisky, his body had not grown better with age.

With a combination of speed and servitude that only the young possess, I was in the kitchen lifting the circle of cloth off the floor, where I then stood by the stove and watched him negotiate the sea of orange before I read the rest of the article. The article was engrossing as it dealt with Boyd's fall from nine years of sobriety, which at that time was about how long Dad had been sober. It would take another ten years before I picked up on Dad's abstinence approach to living, but anyway, that was the first of many times I heard "Boy, have you read Denny Boyd today?"

"The newspaper guy, right?" asked Shelly.

"Yup."

"Well?"

I didn't really want to continue since I knew she wouldn't understand, but somehow I had gotten myself to this point and I had to bring it all out into the open. "I think Pete McMartin smokes during training."

"What? Dave, he probably drinks too. What in the world are you thinking? He's not the new Suzette Meyers, is he?" asked Shelly.

I heard a mocking "Yeah, Suzette Meyers" repeated by the littler one, which threw me into a stuttering "No, no, no. She's a newscaster, and he's a writer."

They both glared at me as if I had just accused them of being a couple of Duchovny's by asking them if they knew anything at all about rain.

I shook my head and said a few more no's before telling them that Suzette Meyers had nothing to do with this. I'll never know why in this family all roads must lead back to a guy's favourite newscaster.

"Well, what's Denny Boyd got to do with all this?" asked Shelly.

So this was where I told her about the tipping point in the training and how it had me on edge. Then I told her about how long and lonely the walking portions were, and how I would review McMartin's weekly column during this time, and how this all had somehow degenerated into convincing myself that Pete McMartin smoked during the walking portions. I mean, with all the walking it was possible—if he smoked, that is, and I had no idea if McMartin did.

So who you gonna ask? Pete McMartin? Yeah, right. He may be the big cheese of asking questions, but I couldn't imagine him actually answering any. It just doesn't work that way. Could former B.C. Lions defensive lineman Nick Hebler take a few snaps? Naw, nothing against the big Hay Baler, but if he switched from defence to offence he would tackle himself. The same with Olympic bronze medallist Harry Jerome. Could he run marathons at the drop of a hat? I don't think so. The sprinter's fast-twitch muscles just wouldn't allow it. So McMartin could make a valiant attempt to surrender his basic instincts by dropping the proverbial felt fedora (you know, the one with the little white press ticket sticking cockeyed out of the band), but he still would not be able to answer my questions about him. To me it was just the fundamentals, or at least that was my twisted justification on that particular day at that particular moment.

So who *are* you gonna ask? Denny Boyd, of course. Boyd's and McMartin's careers overlapped down at the *Vancouver Sun*, and if anyone should know the inside scoop on McMartin it would be the horn blower himself. Boyd had been known to squeeze a bicycle horn at his desk before he sent a finished column off to his editor.

"You leave Denny Boyd alone. He's retired now and doesn't need any of your bogus intrepid reporter baloney," said Shelly. Shelly got up, put the pie in the fridge, took the littler one's hand, and left the kitchen with the final words "And take a shower," which of course was followed up with a "Yeah" from her shadow.

Week 6

Session 1 65 minutes. Run 3 minutes, walk 2 minutes. Do this 13 times. Sunday, February 9, 2003.

I hesitated after locking the door and placing the key in its pouch, which was secured by Velcro to the laces of the right mesh-panelled baby. I put my head back and took a deep breath as I fixed my stare at the tops of a row of thirty-five-year-old fir trees in the neighbours' backyard. The trees were taken as young seedlings from the wilderness, probably the edge of Burns Bog, and were now healthy and fat representations of the species. The fir trees had been topped recently and were now the same height as a row of cedar trees that were in my yard.

As I considered the topping criteria of blending in with the intersecting trees or coming down to some formulated safe height requirement, I realized the true nature of my observation: procrastination. I wasn't breathing heavy, I wasn't sweating, and it seemed that the rain was smacking me harder than usual. There were no fine motor adjustments compensating for the jostling of the eyeballs, no first-step analysis of joint pain, and no double-checking to see if the timer on the watch had been properly activated. I had gotten dressed, initiated the new reduced stretching routine, and stepped outside into the lush multi-hued greenery of the Pacific Northwest, but the scene was static. I wasn't running.

I watched the dark outline of a crow drift down from above and land on one of the fir trees, and a feeling of dread settled into my thighs. I felt incapacitated—as if I couldn't move let alone run between raindrops. I placed my hand over my heart and asked myself, "What have I done?" Here I was about to enter into the biggest day of the Document's schedule, and the pump up the jam was missing. My hand slipped from my chest to my knee as I questioned my decision to reduce the stretching routine. This session was not only the tipping point in moving from more running than walking, at sixty-five minutes it was also the Document's first scheduled session of more than an hour. All told, there would be only four of these peak training sessions over the thirteen-week program.

The wetter I got just standing there flat-footed in the backyard, the more it started to look as if I had inadvertently set in motion all that was needed for a no-go catastrophic event. I gave it a bit more thought, then tore the Velcro straps apart, retrieved the key, and entered the house.

After reviewing the cutbacks, I realized I had plain gone too far, so with renewed resolve I marched through the hallway and entered the bathroom. I had recently developed what I had come to perceive as a secret weapon in my pursuit for an edge in this whole learning to run thing: toothpaste. It wasn't intentional, but I guess with the change in routine I had forgotten to brush my teeth before I left. Actually, it wasn't the teeth that I brushed, it was the tongue. When I was finished, I put a little dab of toothpaste between my cheek and my upper gum, then it was out the door once again and down the driveway. The aspiration of toothpaste down the windpipe and into the lungs was just the ticket for someone who sucked as hard as I did keeping up to the Document's incremental degree of difficulty.

But I gotta tell you, with my suspect right knee, the increased duration, and the fear of actually doing it (you know, running during this session), it all had me pulling way back on the throttle. I focused instead on form throughout the entire sixty-five minutes, which ended up being six loops around the Sungod Track. I held my chin up high, kept the steps short and light, did a few Toller Cranston moves to keep the wrists loose, and made it back relatively unscathed—that is, if you don't include massive exhaustion.

Session 2 50 minutes. Run 3 minutes, walk 2 minutes. Do this 10 times. Tuesday, February 11, 2005.

The euphoria of running more than walking was tempered by my memory of crossing the boulevard on the main entranceway to the Sungod Recreation Centre. It is a five-foot-wide, well-worn shortcut that has all dirt conditions and even curbs to deal with. At one time I had considered the social deviancy of throwing down some bark mulch here, but I now considered the shortcut my initial preparation for going off-track in the real world.

It was the negotiation of the curbs that brought my eyes down to where I witnessed the tender and dainty shuffle of the mesh-panelled babies transporting my bulk through the mud and muck. It was on the second mud fart that I noticed the bright yellow tulips standing sentry off to one side. What was going on here, tiptoeing through the tulips? Visions of Tiny Tim played havoc with the newly printed image of myself becoming a runner. Where was the Bryan Adams power chord, followed up with some loud and raspy declaration of my outstanding athletic achievement? Instead I had to live with the tiddly-wink strumming of a ukulele and the shrill vocals of a performer who appeared to be enjoying everything about himself just a bit too much.

Speed, or rather the lack of it, had been my safeguard against injury and lack of endurance. The low speed limited the effect of my extra weight on each bone-jarring stride, and it also kept hyperventilation at bay, even if I was only two breaths short of seeing double. Now you may want to call me shortsighted, perhaps impatient, or possibly homophobic, but I just had to get the image of Tiny Tim out of my head, and the only way to do that was to turn it up a notch. I had no intention of turning it way up like the day I nearly ran down the dachshund, but I had to attempt something in order to alter the pathos of which I had come to see my training.

146

After the first three-minute run portion on the track, I prepared myself by opening the side vents on the running jacket, which by the way was a serious design improvement over the ragged holes in the lawnmower jacket. I concentrated on good form (such as the arm movements during the walking portion), then launched myself into the second run portion, not with any increased speed over the first run but instead with a degree of obstinacy that even Shelly would find disturbing. I kept my eye on the watch, and when there was fifteen seconds left in the run portion, I lengthened my stride. I practiced this pace change at the end of each of the remaining run portions of the training session, of course while muttering, "Be gone, ye tulip man, be gone," the whole time.

Session 3   55 minutes. Run 3 minutes, walk 2 minutes. Do this 11 times. Thursday, February 13, 2003.

Oh, woe is me. If I had felt a slight soreness after the session-two run, then I was feeling a full level-ten throb after session three. I sat rigid on the edge of the couch, gripping my left knee in an attempt to stabilize myself as I fought the unrelenting pain emanating from the right side of my body. My stare was fixed on the TV as Shelly and Emma alternated the "Are you okay?" question between the two of them, which educed nothing more than a monosyllabic grunt from me since I was grinding my teeth.

I had a hot water bottle on the floor, the underside of my right foot pressing down hard, ensuring complete thermal coverage of the muscles and ligaments from toe to heel. On my right knee I had a frozen bag of peas folded over at the kneecap so I could get side coverage as well. In my right hand wrapped in a towel was a frozen ice pack that I moved in slow motion back and forth on the right calf. I used the commercial breaks to change triage stations from the living room to the kitchen, where I stretched my legs out on the angled painted pile of wood. Once in the kitchen, I could hear snippets of conversation from the living room that ended as I limped back to the heat and ice treatment station.

My reticence set the tone for the quietest night of television we'd ever had—that is, until the TV was turned off and Emma announced that she was going to bed. Then the night became, well, unhinged.

I had gotten up to give Emma a kiss goodnight, then while watching her walk up the stairs to her bedroom, some inexplicable need took hold and made me bend down and pat Rosie, who was curled up in a ball under an end table. The deep knee bend produced a cracking sound that stopped Emma in her tracks, caused Shelly to bolt upright while sinking her clear-coat nails into the arms of the wingback chair, and made the dog yelp before it ran away.

"Are you okay?" was heard one more time that night, this time in unison.

The mere fact that I was able to stand upright without feeling some sort of searing pain was perplexing, and I gave a very milquetoast reply while hoping that more instructive nerve signals were still forthcoming. I did a slow lap around the living room, which gave Emma the reassurance to head upstairs to her room, the dog hot on her heels. Shelly reached for a section of the newspaper when it became obvious that I was zeroing in on the couch. Once seated, I offered up the startling news that I thought the loud noise my lower body had just generated had its origins in my so-called good knee. This news lowered Shelly's newspaper to her chin so that she could peer at me from over the top of her thick, black-framed reading glasses.

"I'd say that you froze that bone good, then snapped it clean in half," said Shelly. She offered to phone 911 once the freezing came out and it became apparent that her Amazing Kreskin powers of foresight were the real deal. Then she went back to reading her newspaper.

My adrenalin spiked as I placed my foot back on the hot water bottle, then placed the frozen peas over my knee. A compassionate wife with soothing words she wasn't. It was more as if an irresistible opportunity had presented itself, and she knew just the button to push while snickering behind the day's headlines. Waves of anxiety rolled over me as I calculated the supply of ice, estimated the ambulance arrival time, and of course prorated the pain factor. Throughout all the math my lips flapped away, with the occasional rustle of section C being the only response.

The topic of my jammering was the latest Pete McMartin column of a couple of days earlier. From heart attacks, to shoes, to bad knees, to McMartin's own math calculations I pretty much recited the entire column without a word or even a blue-eyed glance from Shelly. Then I mentioned the e-mail, and the paper folded inward and was placed aside with machine precision.

"You're not harassing Denny Boyd are you?" asked Shelly.

149

The suddenness of being face to face and needing to switch to the seldom-used answer mode produced a silence that was a bit too long for Shelly's liking, and she was off to the races as she defended the retired columnist's right to privacy. I couldn't get a word in edgewise until Shelly finished up by telling me I was "nothing more than a ballast-belly version of Rachel Marsden."

I'm sure the ice packs receded in size by half from skeletal warming after this accusation of being a serial stalker. I didn't know where to start: Rachel Marsden, Denny Boyd, or Pete McMartin. As much as I wanted to start with Rachel Marsden, I thought it best to ameliorate Shelly's concern for Denny Boyd first, and I reassured her that he wasn't the recipient of the e-mail, it was Pete McMartin. I never did get a good understanding of her protectiveness of Boyd, but the inference didn't go unnoticed that it was all right to poke McMartin. There is something about the mere mention of McMartin's name that is enough to set off a round of stories, usually from early in his career as a sportswriter or during his days as a foreign correspondent.

After Boyd was dealt with, next came Rachel Marsden, who had generated many hours of conversation in this household in the past by being at the centre of two high-profile stalking and harassment controversies. The second controversy arose near the start of my Sun Run training when she was charged with harassing a former Vancouver radio personality. It was this media angle that Shelly had aligned her argument with.

Rachel Marsden's dating mistakes have made the pages of newspapers throughout Greater Vancouver over the years, if only because she wouldn't have it any other way. The judge's comments during Marsden's trial included that she "was extremely extroverted and had some histrionic, attention-seeking traits." I'll say. She sure has generated plenty of attention through water cooler talk, e-mail chatter, and burning phone lines as swim coaches got fired then reinstated and university presidents resigned. In the second controversy she ended up in court, pleading guilty to stalking a former lover.

Years later as I write this memoir, she continues to make headlines as a self-styled political pundit who did not have her contract renewed by the federal Member of Parliament for the North Delta area that I live in. Although the dubious nature of the MP's actions played out publicly, it appears that the only stalking during this incident was by her infamy.

"Now, it's a little over the top to call me a Rachel Marsden after sending one e-mail," I said, withholding comment on her description of my girth.

Shelly is old school. She has only dabbled in this whole e-mail thing of the late twentieth century. So what happens is that she gives e-mails all the formality and careful consideration that she has historically placed in the written letter, which I believe e-mails don't warrant. I know all this from previous conversations about the Y2K millennium bug, where we bounced along a rapid learning curve as we attempted to bring ourselves up to speed on technology, if only to understand why we were going to grind to a halt at the turn of the century.

"Hmm. . . . I just don't see why you need to make this exercise an interactive experience. Can't you just read the paper and then run around the block? Come on, Dave, leave these people alone and just be a normal subscriber," said Shelly.

"He's thinking of doing drugs."

"Oh, good Lord. Like what?"

"Gold injections."

"Oh, for Pete's sake, he's going to use a needle?"

"Hell, I've never even heard of this drug, but it sounds as if he'll shoot it right into his knees."

"Sounds like steroids. We'd better phone your mum," said Shelly.

There could not have been a faster way to stop the conversation dead in its tracks. Phone my mum . . . not a chance. I still get the heebie-jeebies whenever I think back to the last time I talked on the phone to her about steroids. It was the day Ben Johnson's gold medal was stripped from him after he had tested positive for using steroids during the Seoul Olympic Summer Games. Since Mum had been a steroid user for more than thirty years to combat the effects of arthritis, she seemed the natural person to contact for the lowdown on the sprinter's drug of choice. All I did was mention the name Ben Johnson and a low, stone-grinding Scottish accent that I had never heard in all my years resonated over the earpiece. It enunciated every syllable with sinister inflection when it said, "That scunner, he ran a dirty race." Oh, it was nasty, and it left me doing a small bobble-head for the remainder of the long-distance phone call. No, I didn't want to bring up the Ben Johnson conversation. Ever again.

When I reminded Shelly of why I wouldn't be phoning home, she switched the conversation back to the contents of the e-mail. She groaned when I told her I was dispensing advice, then picked up the conversation once again when I mentioned I had invited McMartin out for a little rehabilitation on the soft bark-mulch surface of the Sungod Track.

"You know, with his drug treatments and conditioning that can only be superior to yours, he's going to use you for passing practice," said Shelly.

I hadn't thought of that. In fact, I had only genuine concern for his health, which included wondering if he would be hiding any booze bottles around the track the night before. Then there was the sixty-four thousand dollar question: did he smoke during the walking portions?

"Yep, he's going to humiliate you, that's for sure. There's only one thing to do. You have to phone Waylon and get something better than this gold stuff," said Shelly.

I was shocked by my wife's transition from calling me a serial stalker to entering me into a battle of the performance enhancers. I remember looking into Shelly's eyes for any sign of mischief regarding the incredulous proposal, but all I got was a batting of eyelashes. A first-date queasiness overtook me. Oh, I was feeling vulnerable under her seductive gaze—you know, with my hot water bottle and my ice packs and all—then I thought of Waylon. He of the bulbous physique who softened his bellicose nature by selling Viagra for Canadian Tire money.

I spent the rest of the night thinking about how much Waylon would charge, because really I didn't know if Shelly could read my mind. Or maybe I was talking in my sleep again. But passing (or specifically my lack of passing) was indeed becoming an issue. Late that night, moments before the sandman's arrival, my last thought was that my Canadian Tire money was far too valuable to be spent keeping up with the McMartins of the world.

Week 7

Session 1 60 minutes. Run 4 minutes, walk 2 minutes. Do this 10 times. Saturday, February 15, 2003.

I suppose some would think the number one reason I didn't get on the steroid bandwagon was that I was afraid of the arthritic finger of Winnie the Gram, Emma's grandmother from Winnipeg, reaching out, dialing my number, and taking exception to my training ethics, but that was not the case. I can't even say the number one reason was that performance-enhancing drugs weren't covered by my medical plan. Being afraid of needles or catching a bad case of 'roid rage didn't make the top of the list either.

Of course, all these things plus the incongruous use of my Canadian Tire money were all up there, but the biggest reason was, and I hate to admit it, well, I just wasn't a hero. I know up to this point I'd been shaking the Document in the air with a great deal of sacramental fervour, but the bottom line at that time was that I wasn't going to let this whole training initiative consume my hard-earned common sense and take me down.

It was pretty simple: I am not a thrill seeker or someone who strives for glory, and I haven't been for a long time. This was not a case of testosterone and human growth hormones dipping dangerously past their normal point of decline due to the aging process, it was something I learned many years ago. And it wasn't that Canadian male moment after I realized the Leafs weren't going to draft me. No, it was much earlier than that, even before I knew how to skate. To quote Popeye the Sailor Man, a television figure from the seminal day when the realization set in, "I yam what I yam."

So as I finished the first session of week seven, I bent over on the track and did the now familiar managerial poke of the knee to check for swelling. Everything seemed fine, but when I stood up and started the walk home from the park, I noticed that I wasn't huffing and puffing the way I normally do. I took this as a sure sign of being on cruise control. Oh, I suppose some new level of fitness had to have been attained at this point, but I didn't look at it that way.

Once I entered the back door, of course with my impeccable session-ending timing, I strode into the kitchen and grabbed a bottle of Aspirin from the highest shelf. This was my drug of choice. Cheap and plentiful, but most of all it didn't mask the pain. I wanted to feel the knee. I wanted to be aware of what was stressing it. I wanted to be conscious of exactly where I stood on pulling the plug on this whole initiative. I gotta tell you, the ball-linked metal chain of the plug was wrapped around my hand so tightly that my Document entry that day looked as if it had been scribbled in using my wrong hand.

Right after showering and getting dressed, I stopped the watch at eighty-one minutes. This was the best part of the run because I was able to shave a minute off the estimated total run time for that session. My experience in manufacturing continued to have a hold on me as I included and assessed the set-up time (that is, warm-up exercises) and the take-down time (that is, showering and changing). Call it compulsion—or maybe it was a sign that I was nothing more than a one-trick pony—but intrinsically I knew that if this total run time figure got out of control, my adherence to the Document would be in jeopardy. So after pushing myself for eighty-one minutes, I sat in and lowered the computer chair, raised my right leg onto a higher kitchen chair, placed the bag of frozen peas over my knee, and (at least from a time perspective) it was mission accomplished for the day's training. I had just clicked on the word processor software when the phone rang.

"Dave, skin rash, weakness, sweating, and palpitations are side effects of medicating with gold. You're not injecting behind my back are you?" asked Shelly.

Shelly had taken it upon herself to become the lead medical researcher in the family after I had convinced myself that I needed surgery on my left heel at the beginning of this whole training initiative. Shelly went on to say that gold wasn't a street drug name for anabolic steroids; in fact, it wasn't a steroid at all. Gold was, of all things, gold, or precisely gold salts, and it was one of the original medications used to treat rheumatoid arthritis. It is prescribed less frequently now since new medications have become available.

You know, being informed and all is a very good thing, but after Shelly hung up I felt a sense of relief by the fact that McMartin wasn't about to embark on some deviant trail that surely would lead to the Hastings Street skid row. It didn't take long, though, before my head was on the table and I was banging my fist, causing Dad's old dictionary to fall to the floor and split open the frozen peas, which had fallen from my knee seconds earlier.

No, I wasn't despondent over not being able to open a paragraph; in fact, I was in full open remorse for having done just that. Shelly had been right. Oh why, oh why had I e-mailed McMartin? It wasn't as if I hadn't put pen to paper for a corporation or a columnist in the past, but there's the rub—I'd always written a letter. How many letters on the day after being written had I walked to the garbage can instead of the postal box? I figured it was probably in the fifty-fifty range, but my e-mails ran flat out at a 100 percent send rate.

Just before the situation deteriorated to sobbing cries of "Don't pass me, again," I calmed myself with thoughts of how many e-mails someone like McMartin would get. I figured twenty for the column, a reasonable number I thought for a non-political health and fitness piece.

I'm sure his work regarding the teachers' union goes exponentially off the charts. Then there would be e-mails from sources and leads for all his other stories on the go, plus some spam and of course the normal deluge from his no-doubt seething and irate editor, so I figured I was safe. You know, my little e-mail would get lost in the mix.

When I felt the edges of this stress begin to lift, I bent over and picked up Dad's dictionary. My eyes fixed on a smattering of peas that the book had liberated when it fell, then as if cued by Poh-Poh herself, my mind drifted back to Dad's kitchen table. For years I had watched him write letters at that table overlooking the daily life of a West End back lane. Conversations and a young assumptive mind led me to believe that he was writing to his friends. But now, after Shelly's accusation that I was nothing more than a Rachel Marsden, it occurred to me that maybe, just maybe, this stalker business ran in the family.

I placed the dictionary before me and opened it up to a page that was anointed with my father's handwriting in blue ink, a math calculation of all things. Could it be that he was writing to Denny Boyd? Naw, the thought was preposterous. After a moment it didn't seem so out there once I factored in the key feature that they were both big alcoholics.

My friend Lenny the boxer, whom I have given the ring name of "Shake and Bake," always questions my use of this moniker. I suppose he just refuses to accept the truth behind it. The "Shake and Bake" story is that whenever he loses, which is more often than not, there is always a point when I can see his eyes cross and a small tremble take hold, then I know it's just a matter of time before he's done like dinner.

Anyway, Lenny also questions my use of the term "big alcoholics." So after many failed attempts to give big alcoholic some sort of dictionary meaning, I'd come to giving it a metaphorical response, that being reporter-at-large Denny Boyd. This media angle finally satisfied Lenny, whose claim to fame by the way doesn't come from inside the ring but from standing outside of it, with one arm on the apron and the other gesticulating wildly while articulating his thoughts on a boxer's life during an interview with Suzette "Best Hands" Meyers. Yes, both Lenny and I have voted her "Best Hands" in the TV Personality category. This Lenny is a one-man storm; poor woman probably thought she was going to take a roundhouse while rebuffing haymakers with her ever-present steno notepad.

I was assessing the long-term sobriety angle between the two big alcoholics when the ghost of Jack Wasserman floated ominously across the flickering blank page on the computer screen. By my estimation, Denny earned a big portion of the metaphor in 1968 when he took over the *Vancouver Sun* saloon column. This was when he followed in fellow *Sun* reporter Jack Wasserman's footsteps by dropping into nightclubs all night long. It was when I put together a timeline on Wasserman that I started to get goosebumps. You see, Granddad was a jewellery shopkeeper at Granville and Georgia, smack in the middle of Wasserman's beat, right at the height of the reporter's heyday. I just can't see how those two never met. After all they were, well, for fear of overusing the phrase, big alcoholics. They both were reputed to like their booze—a lot. So this was the genesis of my theory on multi-generational stalking that haunts me to this very day.

I turned off the computer and cursed Rachel Marsden. I didn't need this whole stalking thing getting in the way of my training. And as for McMartin, just to be on the safe side I told Shelly and the littler one to tell anyone who phoned for me that I was out of the country. A couple of days later I overheard Emma answer the phone then say that her dad was "out of it" before promptly hanging up.

Session 2 54 minutes. Run 4 minutes, walk 2 minutes. Do this 9 times. Monday, February 17, 2003.

In Carol Shields's *The Stone Diaries*, far and away my favourite aspect of the novel is the opening setting. Now I don't want to take anything away from the plot, which starts out in bizarre fashion, nor is it my intention to damn the characters with faint praise, but the setting is what captivated me. There are a few reasons for this, the first being that I was born and raised in the Winnipeg area, so I have firsthand knowledge of the locale.

The opening setting is actually just outside of Winnipeg around the town of Tyndall, where beautiful dolomite limestone is quarried. This Tyndall Stone, which at the time I thought every city had access to, is prevalent throughout Winnipeg in the construction of its churches and older mansions. It wasn't until I began to visit distant cities that I became aware of the fact that not all cities grew from solid off-white foundations that firmly ensconced the local history. Tyndall Stone is truly a material of affirmation, with the Manitoba Legislative Building serving as the mineral's finest display. *The Stone Diaries* opens in the year 1905, which brings me to the main reason the setting took such a hold of me. My Hutchinson ancestors had come to Canada nine years earlier, and of course where did they settle? Just outside Winnipeg.

When my great granddad John Hutchinson of Red Hill, County Caven, Northern Ireland, immigrated to Canada with his wife Sarah Jane, it was to make a better life for themselves. They were leaving behind famine, civil unrest, and the risk of being shipped out to the British West Indies as slaves when they chose the frigid winters and boiling summers of the Canadian prairies. Now this is where Carol Shields's description of the Goodwill family and her vivid depiction of their sustenance tugged on my heartstrings. As I read about the Goodwills, I could envision the Hutchinsons and the Clouters (Sarah Jane's family) living down the street. I'll never forget the sentiment that welled within me while reading those opening chapters; it was truly a remarkable experience.

The protagonist in *The Stone Diaries* is not Cuyler Goodwill but his daughter Daisy. My choice of Cuyler as a focal point is a testament to Carol Shields's authoritative ability to create depth and understanding beyond the story's main character. The same can be said about Wayson Choy's Poh-Poh. These stirring characters have the ability to inspire, enlighten, and enchant as their charisma exudes from the pages, creating an aura of literary wonder for the reader.

Ten years into retirement, Cuyler Goodwill was lying on the soft green grass before his partially completed scaled model of Egypt's Great Pyramid. When finished, he would have cut and placed two million three-eighth-inch square pieces of stone that he had collected from around the world. At that moment in time, with the warmth of the sun upon his face, his thoughts weren't on finishing, however; they were on bringing an abrupt halt to the project. The master stonecutter's dilemma was that his monument at the quarter completion point was out of plumb. This information was nothing short of catastrophic; if he continued, the situation would only get worse, with the final result of a lopsided pyramid being unacceptable. Cuyler's only options were to either stop or start over again.

I stood at the end of the driveway, put my hands on my hips, and looked towards the willow tree on the corner. There was no need to look at my right knee, there was no need to give it a poke, there was no need to ask the gas-meter reader walking by for a quick opinion. It looked fine, and I knew that from the intense scrutiny I had given it since my first waking moment that morning. It may not have looked swollen, but it felt mushy—like mashed potatoes that had become liquefied—with all the various cartilage, ligaments, bone, and bursae now swimming in this murky white fluid even as I stood rigidly facing the route to the Sungod Track.

I thought of Cuyler, I thought of the Document, I thought of knee replacement surgery, then I heard the beep from my wristwatch and with a jolt I pressed on. Test step, test step, then at the minute and a half mark I transitioned from a slow run to walking. I had not known when that transition point was going to take place; all I had known was that I wasn't going to run the full four minutes. Prudence, convention, and common sense had won the inner battle for self-preservation.

Shortly after waking, I had resigned myself to the fact that this would be the inglorious and shameful day that I would move away from the literal interpretation of the Document. I had fumbled through the coffee-making process, mindlessly flipped through the newspaper, then drifted alongside Emma in silence during the walk to school. My cherished ideals, principles, and practices and the standards that they produced were now under assault, and although my remedial corrective action had merit, I was crestfallen. Whereas Cuyler's choice was to bring his project to a halt, I chose to start over. Well, almost. This is where the minute and a half of running came in. I didn't know what the run numbers would be, but the plan was to dig back into the Document and run for a comfortable length of time, then extend the walking portion to bring it up to the stated length of time for week seven, session two.

During all the extra walking, I spent an inordinate amount of time looking over my shoulder. You know, just to be on the lookout for McMartin should he pick today, the most inopportune of days, to jaunt by, twisting and teasing me in the swell of his scarf.

.

Session 3 54 minutes. Run 4 minutes, walk 2 minutes. Do this 9 times. Wednesday, February 19, 2003.

"Hey, Rocketman, get over here." Shelly rarely missed an opportunity to laugh at my expense. So as I finished the last session of week seven, she had curled her legs up underneath herself while sitting at one end of the couch, finger-combed her locks in an enticing fashion, and mocked my appearance at the back door. She was imitating (rather well, I must say) a pain reliever commercial on television in which a temptress calls out to her main squeeze, who has just staggered into their abode in obvious pain while wearing sweaty running gear.

In fact, I had played my role rather well, or I should say rather too well. The whole reduced running time aspect of the previous session and the ensuing defeated shuffle produced a psychological floundering that only Emma's Barbie collection was able to rectify. While changing into my running gear, I knew I wouldn't be doing the reduced run again, but I wasn't exactly brimming with confidence—or at least I wasn't until Barbie spoke to me.

I had been leaning over a large toybox, brimming with Barbie dolls and paraphernalia, to get my running shirt from the closet when a disembodied voice said, "I love your hair." It gave me a start (you know, being in the darkness of the closet and all), but I eventually figured that my right knee had pressed against the toybox, so I kneed the box again and it said, "I love your outfit. You look cool." It was all way too unexpected and way too enjoyable, so with one hand on the hanger for support, I thrust my knee into it again and again and again: "You look awesome." "It's fun to be with you." "You look hip."

I stared into the box but couldn't determine what doll or gadget was befriending me, but that didn't stop me from continuing the mollycoddling of my self-esteem. All told, there were sixteen different uplifting expressions that sent me down the driveway on a high, with no reservations or self-checks in place whatsoever. So that's my explanation for the slight pull in my right thigh that resulted in a bit of a limp, which set the scenario for Shelly's greeting, and I'm sticking to it.

All in all it was a huge relief to be finished with week seven. Deviating from the Document had been spiritually devastating, but if truth be told it would have paled in comparison to the physical destruction that I felt would have been imminent if I hadn't.

Week 8

Session 1 60 minutes. Run 5 minutes, walk 1 minute. Do this 10 times. Saturday, February 22, 2003.

I lifted a roll and jabbed my thumb down until the nail was immersed. Not satisfied, I twisted my torso and stabbed my thumb into a second roll. This time the cuticle was still exposed, even after having the thumb bottom out and giving it a few extra skin-burning twists. It was the second roll that lifted my spirits, with its density of one hundred knots per square inch. Having met my prescribed criteria of comfort, I threw the carpet roll over my shoulder, turned out the light, and exited the small arid confines of the attic.

Shelly rotates the household area rugs between accenting various rooms and taking up storage space whenever the mood strikes her. Some of the rugs I don't see for years, which always makes their unrolling a big event. With the extra weight of the rug, the sound of my footsteps made me want to roar, "Fe fi fo fum!" but I took pity on the dog and kept the puerile thoughts and boorish expression to myself.

Once down the stairs I crossed through the living room, then unrolled the rug in the hallway where I did my warm-up exercises. As soon as I had rolled out the training aid, I put it to use by getting flat on my back. I placed a leg up on the interior doorway wall, stretched my hamstring, and basked in the sensation of being held aloft by each of the hand-knotted, cut-pile strands of wool.

Shelly walked in after her day at work, saw me flat out on the area rug, and said, "Oh." She then stepped over me and said, "Oh." Really, at that point I would have preferred an "oh" followed by a "baby, baby, oh baby, baby," one hand on a gyrating hip and the other waving her sweater over her head, but so much for the male fantasy. All I got were a few more "ohs" as she stepped around and over my roly-poly mass, drinking in the different angles, then said, "At least you're not kissing it this time."

The area rug was the perfect workout mat, and with Shelly home to look after Emma, I finished my exercises, got dressed, and hit the Sungod Track.

I started feeling a touch uncomfortable once I reached the portion of the track parallel to the boulevard along the east entrance driveway. This was the third day after my last run, and I was feeling the effects of that extra day off big time. The burning sensation in my lungs was such that the mashed-potato syndrome associated with my right knee had become a moot point as I struggled for existence in the seemingly oxygen-deficient park. Pit zippers came down, followed by a quick Toller Cranston hand roll for stress relief, then the left arm came up for a time check. The grunt generated after determining I was not yet halfway to the Document's promised nirvana of one minute walking coincided with a small rustling in the undergrowth on my right. I didn't flinch as I kept my eyes fixed on the watch as it counted up to the five-minute mark.

I put my arm down as I navigated the crosswalk at 111th Street, which demarks the point in the track where the bottom of its L shape turns up northward to the top of the L. It was here, while under the most physically taxing of circumstances, that the sweat from my brow forever etched into my eyes the image of a massive vertical peak. The terror of this realization brought the watch back up to see if there was any civil way around the impending wretched incline of despair—like was the run portion of this interminable segment up yet? Because of the varying lengths of the Document's run and walk portions in each training session, I had never had to run up this portion of the Sungod Track before, but now the confluence of track design and the Sun Run program was going to test my mettle.

I brought my arm down, lifted my chin up to straighten and shorten the respiratory pathway, then saw another first as I began the ascension: a peak-a-boo view of the North Shore's Seymour Mountain that lasted maybe ten steps before it disappeared behind a row of fir trees. I continued to keep my chin up, downloading oxygen in the most efficient manner possible, and shortened my already stunted stride as I concentrated on the image of the mountain. The more my lungs hurt, the higher I lifted my chin, until the roll of fat on the back of my neck started to hurt as well.

To check the time while in this running posture, I needed to hold my hand in full extension well over my head. The hand and LCD watch came down with the abruptness of a race-ending checkered flag the second the run portion was over. This gave me the necessary two-handed stabilization to hunch over my knees. After the prerequisite emergency breaths, I saw a clump of five alder trees, their presence signalling that I was at the top of the hill.

I stood up and took a few steps, then almost went for a tumble. Although the ascension is long and gradual, the drop-off from the top of the hill is steep and dramatic. I ended up bumping along the drop-off as if going down a set of stairs after a ringing phone. At the bottom I looked over my shoulder at my accomplishment and was amazed—not at the size of the hill but at how I had never considered it a hill before.

During the one-minute walking portion, I surveyed the entire track and saw that the hill was actually a man-made berm and that there were two of them, one at each end of the park. I can only surmise that, back when they first built the pool and the ice rink facilities, for cost reasons they had simply pushed the excavated earth to each end of the work site. Years later, as the bark mulch was laid around the perimeter of the park, the berms inadvertently added a new dimension: hill climbing. I thanked my lucky stars when I later filled out the log portion of the Document that I had not run the entire length of Berm's Peak last week. With my knee and all, who knows if the whole training initiative would have given up the ghost had I done the peak in week seven?

I also wrote that my right knee was a bit better, then I added, "Did it!" *Did it* had nothing to do with my knee, and it certainly wasn't about mustering up the courage to do steroids, nor was it about passing another runner on the track (I wish). *Did it* had everything to do with recovery. Forget the Denny Boyd angle, *did it* was about walking for one minute. You see up to this point, the Document had been lobbing thirty-second chunks off the walking portions whenever it changed, but in week eight there was a drastic one-minute drop-off that had me shaking in my mesh-panelled babies. I wondered at that time if my poor performance in the previous week had something to do with my analysis of this drop-off and the resulting anxiety I had brought upon myself.

My faith in the Document during this period had been severely tested, so I think the exclamation mark was more for its benefit, since my mere completion of the session reaffirmed that the Document was charting a proper course. Praise the Document and grab a dry towel.

Session 2 48 minutes. Run 5 minutes, walk 1 minute. Do this 8 times. Monday, February 24, 2003.

I had not yet replaced the cap on the pen after filling out the log for session one when Shelly pulled a chair out of her way and stood at the opposite end of the kitchen's harvest table, enabling her under-five-foot frame to bear down on me. I looked up and felt great gobs of guilt at using a dishtowel to wipe the sweat off my brow.

But before any apology could be sputtered, Shelly said, "Tell me what it says."

Oh, boy. Sensing I was in trouble but not knowing what for, I blurted out, "Did it!"

Shelly gave me a smirk that rivalled Pete McMartin's, gave her head a barely perceptible shake, then said, "Keep your did its to yourself. What does that piece of paper say?"

The pen rattled as I tossed it aside, and my chairback could be heard sliding along the wall in my haste to stand and hand the Document across the table. I was having difficulty comprehending her implication, so as I leaned over the table I asked, "You want to run?"

Shelly held her hands up over her head at the offering, as if afraid of being burned. "Sit down, Hutchinson. I said tell me what it says."

I sat back down and held the Document with one hand while I gripped the edge of the table with the other. Shelly continued to talk, but my hearing had shut off. I was dumbfounded. My wife was non-athletic. She had no history of playing sports while growing up in Vancouver's West End, none whatsoever. My vision of her participation in phys. ed. while going to King George High School is one of lounging through the various coffee houses on Denman Street. Of course this is a testosterone-driven vision that includes the prerequisite wardrobe of a push-up bra, leopard-skin tights, and those black, pointy cats-eye glasses. Shelly is completely at my mercy when I throw a dirty sock at her because she can't catch, hockey sticks are only good for removing cobwebs in high places, and I'd never seen her run across the street.

I continued to drift along in my own thoughts, working on the best-case scenario of Shelly running the Sun Run 2003 at my side. The math calculations were fast and furious as I pro-rated, cut corners, and planned an all-out training regimen that would get her to the starting line. I was double-checking some kilometre-to-mile conversions just to make Shelly feel comfortable during my presentation, when a deep, husky, and obviously theatrical voice brought me back to my wife standing at the head of the table.

"Hutchinson, Hutchinson, Hutchinson, you know what I mean? I am not running in the Sun Run." She was playing a bit-part tough-guy character from a manuscript of mine that she had read years earlier. The tables had turned, and it was Shelly who was making me feel comfortable, and once she saw me smiling she continued. "I knew that would warm the cockles of your heart. Now tell me, what does it say."

"Run thirty seconds."

"Oh."

I got up from the table, told Emma in the next room that we were moving out, then explained to Shelly that we were going shoe shopping. I got zero resistance. The three of us drove to the second-closest sporting goods store to our house. I couldn't go to the nearest one—time had not yet healed that nasty piece of shopping. Once inside, we sat with Shelly in front of the great wall of shoes until a sales representative engaged us. With this part of the mission accomplished, Emma and I circumvented the inevitable retail battle fatigue and cut out to the neighbouring coffeehouse to await Shelly's return, when we would admire the shopper's spoils.

I had decided I was not going to read the Document to Shelly, and of course for whatever reason she wasn't even going to pick it up. Instead, my plan was to show her how to run, so for week eight, session two Shelly joined me. Now I had no intention of going backwards in the program again, but Shelly's unexpected involvement provided the opportunity to do so. I found the prospect of running thirty seconds intriguing because the reduced run time last week had proved so beneficial to my knee that I thought it would be so again. I also just wanted to experience the thirty-second sensation one more time. The pain and agony of that first day continued to haunt me, and now I could verify the authenticity of that memory.

During the hamstring portion of the warm-up exercises, I showed Shelly how to do the stretches herself by using the doorway on an interior wall. (The football move was still banned, so I couldn't hold her leg for her.) It was while admiring the angle of her stretch and the ease with which she seemed to accomplish it that I noticed she had on a different pair of runners. When I inquired as to whether I was losing my mind in regard to the runners, she replied that she exchanged the other pair earlier in the day. Oh, I instantly felt weak. All I could think of was Poh-Poh and what she would say about this apparent repeat of recent history. The excitement and energy of the training session drained unabated even after Shelly said, "It's no big deal, Dave. I did what you told me to do, and after wearing them around the house for a day I decide to exchange them."

Being shell-shocked and all I didn't say a word as we walked to the Sungod Track. At the track I lifted my wrist, reset the timer on the watch, and said, "Go"—at which point we proceeded to body slam each other. Shelly had gone clockwise, and I had gone counter-clockwise.

An old-fashioned, lovely evening in the park, husband–wife argument ensued as we faced each other and debated which direction we were going to run around the track. Well, I lost the argument big time, and there was a very good reason why. There is some kind of strange phenomenon concerning direction of movement and the Sungod Track. For some inexplicable reason, walkers tend to go clockwise around the track, while runners use it counter-clockwise. I don't know why this is, but even I use the track this way, and this is where Shelly won out. The crux of her argument was that we had used the track many times over the years, always going clockwise. "Why would we go counter-clockwise today?"

With open-mouthed wonder at losing to the precedent-based argument, stymied at running a measly thirty seconds, and fixated on whether Shelly's Achilles heel would give out on her, our first show-and-tell training session together was completed. While doing the dinner dishes with Shelly, I peppered her with questions about her health. How's your heel, how's your knee, how's your back, how was your breathing? I revisited the heel again and again each time, probing from a different angle, not believing one feel-good word of what I was hearing.

About halfway through the dishes, I sat down with my drying towel while Shelly kept her hands busy in the dishwater. This produced a protracted silence. The view I had was of her back, which I fixed my eyes upon as I reviewed the entire training session one more time. Then all elbow movement, all washing sounds, and the gentle swaying of her hair stopped, and she spoke in a soft voice without turning away from her window view of the neighbours' cedar trees.

"Dave," said Shelly with an ominous hesitation that made me thankful I was sitting down. "Dave, do you think you could run a little faster?"

What was going on here? Some non-athlete breezing through the first Sun Run session, then telling her embarrassment of a husband, who back in the day used to paint his cleats gold—have I mentioned that before?—to pick up the pace. I suppose these could have been interpreted as fighting words, but if the truth be told, Shelly could have said almost anything, including, "Dave, you're a lousy lover," as long as she didn't say, "Dave, I quit."

My reply was, "Yes, Shell, and you done good. You know what I mean."

Session 3 54 minutes. Run 5 minutes, walk 1 minute. Do this 9 times. Wednesday, February 26, 2003.

I charged hard across the Sungod Track's 111th Street crosswalk, which brought me to the start of the Berm's Peak ascension. Of course, such superfluous bursts of energy were not a normal part of my routine, but it was one of those life-saving moments. You see, this crosswalk has a particular quirk to it in that vehicles do not slow down in their approach; in fact, they often accelerate through it. My usual practice for this crosswalk was to gear way down if I saw an oncoming vehicle so that it didn't need to stop for me. But I guess on this day I was concerned about the start of Berm's Peak and entered the crosswalk unprepared. When I determined that the vehicle was speeding up, it forced me into the hard charge, or maybe the expression "did a quick two-step" would be more apt.

When I first started running the Sungod Track, I thought this crosswalk phenomenon was another example of the differences between urban drivers and their suburban counterparts, with the suburban drivers being much less tolerant of pedestrians. Then, after witnessing the drivers' heads bobble under accelerative forces as they zoomed past me a few times, I began to think it was all about me. I remember thinking at the time that I could be provoking them with my red jacket cum target and that I should stop all Toller Cranston arm movements leading up to the crosswalk for fear that this could be seen as inciting the game-on mentality.

Later that training session, I figured out that it wasn't about me, but about a speed hump. When a driver catches sight of a pedestrian entering the crosswalk, if he stops before the speed hump, the car ends up being too far back; conversely the car ends up too far forward if the driver stops after the hump, and I've never seen anyone perch a vehicle on the three foot wide hump itself. This just doesn't seem to be done in these parts. Maybe the drivers are afraid of some kind of undercarriage damage if they stop mid-hump, but they certainly aren't afraid of upper vertebra damage as they ride that hump competitively in order to beat me through the crosswalk.

Now, I'm not going to get into Pete McMartin territory and say that my crosswalk showdown was with a yummy mummy cruising in an SUV, but I guess I could only be so lucky (you know, with the extra road clearance and all if I ever did get hit). This particular encounter was with a young lad rocking by in a two-door Japanese import whose polished rims could be seen reflecting on the wet roadway. McMartin generated some hoopla a few years ago when in one of his columns he referred to the women of Twasassen, his area of residence, as yummy mummies who drove British-made Land Rovers along palm-treed boulevards. Comparatively, North Delta's McKitrick Park boulevard leading to the Sungod Recreation Centre has mostly pine trees with North American minivans parked under them.

The energy expenditure from going through the crosswalk left me running on fumes for the entire Berm's Peak ascension. It felt as if I was back on my first day of training, where I held my breath and muscled my way through the session. For the one-minute walking portion after Berm's Peak, I pulled over to the side of the trail and stretched my calf muscles using the smooth edge of a small boulder. I placed my head back all the way, causing sweat to dribble down my neck, then I leaned as far forward over my knee as I could get. The position and humidity produced by the exercise gave my skin a greasy, viscous snail feel, but all wetness aside, it made for a respiratory recovery that could only be described as miraculous.

After the stretching, which much to my surprise offered little resistance, I brought my head up and got in about ten seconds of walking before it was time to run again. The very second that the walk portion was over, my lower legs and the mesh-panelled babies sprung into action without any coaxing whatsoever. There were a few large air gasps, probably from the suddenness of it all, but basically it felt as if my body was in complete control and all my mind had to do was interpret the LED readout on the watch.

At the end of the training session, Shelly met me in the driveway with the stopwatch instead of her reading glasses dangling around her neck and my wallet and car keys in her hand. "Okay, my turn," said Shelly as she handed me my stuff and got in her vehicle, where Emma and Rosie were waiting. As per the plan, I was to drive her to the Sungod Track and keep an eye on her while she trained in the shadows of the late winter evening. I did not want to risk losing any training gains by going backwards in the program again, but I wasn't all that enthused about Shelly running through the park by herself in the low light conditions.

After we parked in the Sungod lot, beeps and clicks emanated from the vehicle's interior. At the conclusion of the stopwatch demonstration, Shelly slipped off her seat and exited through the open door. Faster than I could say "Emma, forward troop movement," the door was opened wide again and Shelly asked, "What does it say?" *It* being the Document, whose bent edges and perspiration-smudged passages Shelly refused to hold in her pampered hands. I took immense pleasure in repeating my favourite portion of the Document: "Run thirty seconds."

I watched her run off, but instead of redeploying Emma and the dog, I started the vehicle and put it in gear. I had to turn around because, holy smokes, she was running counter-clockwise.

The reorientation of my view of Shelly on the track placed the vehicle ninety degrees to the speed hump on the Berm's Peak ascension. We were so close to the track that Shelly had to take only two steps out of her way to give me a high-five—you know, if she should pick up on such sis-boom-bah behaviour. Really, after directional changes, could end-of-training-session water-barrel-tossing over an obnoxious husband's head be far behind? Yes, obnoxious, but I couldn't help myself, being so close to the track and all. So each time Shelly passed by, I rolled down the window and the family gave her some encouragement. In retrospect, maybe the neighbourhood could have done without the honking, but a quick and polite Queen's wave just didn't seem appropriate for such a feat coming from someone who had never run before in her life.

Later that night, Shelly and I talked about this directional thing. Although we hadn't discussed it since our initial confrontation, the possibility that I had been exerting pressure in some passive way over the last couple of days didn't sit well with me. We've been married many years, so you must know that this wasn't the first time I'd heard over the course of a conversation that I had a tendency to take all the fun out of things. Spirit smotherers such as having one rule too many, regulations that are beyond reason, and a specification or two that are just not necessary in the Hutchinson household. Shelly then added that I should "chill out" in this instance because she had based her actions on her own field research. Apparently she had stopped by the North Delta High School track on her way home from work the last couple of days and took note that 100 percent of the facilities' participants used the track in a counter-clockwise fashion. Sensing that I was off the hook, I declared "Enough said" and we went to bed.

I was drifting off towards sleep, feeling that I had a better understanding of why Shelly refused to touch the Document, when the nightmare slide show kicked in, creating a boiling bilious sensation that pushed hard against my lower drawstring. The still-frame image that sat rigid in the viewfinder of my mind was of a stopped vehicle. Yes, it was on the hump, and yes, it had stopped for Shelly as she crossed the 111th Street crosswalk. I knew then that this whole crosswalk thing really was about me and those darn bobble heads. To say that I slept poorly that night would be an understatement.

Week 9

Session 1
63 minutes. Run 7 minutes, walk 2 minutes. Do this 7 times. Friday, February 28, 2003.

I wish I could say I was all fired up for this training session because of its total time of more than sixty minutes, but I can't. It just seemed I was afraid to confront the challenges head on and instead found some other distraction to disassociate myself from the rigours of following the Document. For the first portion of this training session, that is exactly what I did as I assessed my adherence to the Document.

I plotted the total training times of each session on a mental graph as I made my way around the soft Sungod Track from one berm to another, alternating between alder canopies, the long shadows provided by fir trees, and the bright blue sky. Week one started off at thirty-five minutes, then moved it up a notch to forty minutes. Week two started off at forty-five minutes, then backed off to forty minutes. The Document's total run times took shape on the mental graph until it resembled a stock market graph. Or at least it resembled a stock market graph that I would have liked to have bought shares in on day one. It went up a bit then came down a bit. Then it would jag back up and dip a bit. The end result was a net gain on each upward spike, which resulted in an upward trend for the overall course of the information plotted to that date.

The graph contained two asterisks, denoting that I had put in the total time but had walked most of those sessions. As I looked at the two pull-back sessions, it visually affirmed what I had felt all along: I had done the right thing. Having amused then pleased myself by manipulating the statistics to meet my emotive needs, I moved on to Shelly's math calculations. There was nothing spontaneous about her beginning to train when she did. By choosing to start when she did, she ensured that there would not be sufficient time to complete the training regimen before the start of the Sun Run.

If I knew Shelly, the timing also had something to do with not accumulating stress. Just the normal things in life like working and raising a family were enough; adding a timeline with an absolute unknown physical component to it just wasn't necessary. But hey, she was participating, and this had me admiring her for being such a smooth calculator as I completed the remainder of the training session.

Although I was tired because of the peak training time, I was able to complete the session in a relatively easy manner because the walk time had been increased to two minutes. This was the last week for walking two minutes, and I made sure that I squeezed every last micro-second out of them. Even at this stage in the training, I did not consider myself a runner. In fact, because I was so concerned about my physical well-being, I didn't know if it was possible to become one. There is no doubt that I had developed performance anxiety, and the proof of this was my fixation on the late entry date for Sun Run registration.

Session 2 54 minutes. Run 7 minutes, walk 2 minutes. Do this 6 times. Monday March 3, 2003.

"There's a runner."

This expression had become the new family catchphrase while driving about the neighbourhood. It was a significant upgrade from "Punch buggy, no return." More often than not, a vociferous outcry would reveal the runner's presence when he was nothing more than a distant and tiny dancing ball of reflective light. The reflective material of either glass beads or metallic particles seems to be sewn into the shoes, pants, gloves, and jackets of pretty much every runner who has an evening run routine.

The call had gone out, and we were watching the approaching dancing ball stretch out into bobbing lines, which moments later developed the soft, tapered edges of a runner's profile emerging from the infinite black background of a quiet suburban side street. Facial features were always the last aspect to be illuminated by the vehicle's lights, giving them the shortest time span of being visible.

"Hey, that's Nancy," said Emma.

I didn't get a look at her because I was driving, but more often than not I was never able to see anyone who was running at night unless she happened to be running under a streetlight as we passed each other. Instinctively I looked in the rear-view mirror, but I couldn't find the rhythmic reflective form. Shelly and I were taking Emma to Brownies when we saw Nancy, who had dropped her daughter off with the Brownie leaders and was doing her training run in the immediate neighbourhood.

As a Vancouver Sun Run Team Leader for North Delta, Nancy trained once per week out of the Sungod Recreation Centre. She had told me in previous curbside chats (in between my persistent, single-minded, and single question of "Where do you run?") that a smaller portion of the Sun Run training group runs together on a second day and that she runs solo for the week's third day of training. Talk about pressure. I was kind of hoping that the powerbabe down the street would have just plain quit or maybe come down with some sort of orthotic syndrome du jour, forcing her out of the training, but that hadn't happened yet.

Although my resolve to continue was as strong on this day as it had been on day one, I remember thinking that it would have been nice to have a built-in "out." You know, just in case things got a little hairy once this whole walk portion of the training was over and done with. As it was, I willingly suited up three times a week, but it was accomplished with an equal measure of trepidation.

After dropping Emma off at Brownies, Shelly and I drove over to the Sungod Track for a training run. We staggered our running positions on the Sungod Track so I could keep an eye on her while we each completed our own training sessions. This fresh approach produced the opportunity to work on my speed as I chased Shelly down throughout the session. I was surprised that it took almost the entire fifty-four minutes for me to catch up to her, as I would close in only to lose most of those gains during the two-minute walking portions of the session.

We drove back to the Brownie meeting, and while we waited for Emma, I continued my single-minded and single-question inquisition of Nancy. "So, where did you run?" By my estimation at that time, there were no flat routes to run in North Delta. Where once upon a time, in some vehicle-dependent pre–Sun Run training life, I had thought that North Delta was positively flat, it certainly wasn't the case as I talked to Nancy. My most recent land surveys while walking Emma to school—and of course the valuable information gleaned by my monotonous interviewing technique—suggested that life was all uphill outside the cozy confines of the Sungod Track. Nancy loathed the hill work so much that I became nauseated while listening to her training stories, and as I stood there I found myself longing for the comfortable non-athletic hours of warm amplifier tubes and sloppy stacks of CDs to listen to, for the rest of time.

On the drive home, I thought of a better and physically brave alternative: the New Year's Day Polar Bear Swim. I had read about individuals obtaining official accreditation for participating in the swim from the event organizers, even when they did the swim while on vacation outside the country or in spite of whatever their biggest problem was on that day. So anyway, it got me thinking that maybe I could do the same thing for the Sun Run. You know, just run it solo at the Sungod Track in McKitrick Park. Obviously I am not a real social butterfly, and since the Sun Run billed itself as a large social event of more than forty-five thousand people, well you know they wouldn't miss me. I figured this angle deserved a bit more attention over the next couple of days.

As I filled out the training log that night, it occurred to me that I might have unwittingly passed the point of no return. The point of no return scared the dickens out of me because I did not feel like a runner, and if that was the case, what in the world had I become? And what was I doing three times a week in the park? I put the pen down and cursed myself for not planning some sort of easy out in this whole running initiative.

Session 3 50 minutes. Run 8 minutes, walk 2 minutes. Do this 5 times. Thursday, March 6, 2005.

From an environmental perspective, my Sun Run training to date had been accomplished under typical winter conditions for the Greater Vancouver area. This means no snow and lots of rain. Of course, accompanying the rain was a horizon-to-horizon overcast sky that relegated the sun to some sort of low-wattage frosted light bulb status. The decorative lighting aspect of the season changed on this day, though, with a certain degree of intensity, which opened up a whole new world of taste and smell.

I first noticed the taste while licking my fingertips. I'm a fingertip licker from way back—it's sports related, you see. A quick fingertip lick, catch the football. Another self-congratulatory fingertip lick for catching it, double licks if it was a first down, then repeat the cycle over again. No one ever commented on it at the time, but they sure did on the Toller Cranston hand roll, which many teammates found perplexing. You see, this was where the move first became incorporated. Lick the fingertips, then place the palms face down in front of the torso—oh, about waist high—then bring them up and over and have the ball land simultaneously in the exposed palms and outstretched fingers. It was all a timing and rhythm thing, with a touch of superstition thrown into the mix for good measure. The move even had a slightly altered version for cradling balls thrown high over my head, but it worked best for digging balls out of the dirt.

The Toller Cranston hand roll and its accomplice, the fingertip lick, became synonymous with getting the job done. So it wasn't all that surprising that while under the physical stress of ascending Berm's Peak I reverted back to the old comfort zone, but I can't ever remember it tasting as it did that day. Wow, the taste of anchovies made me regret ever learning three-down football. The first lick was merely shocking, then as I came to realize that I had produced the concentrated and foul form of the crystalline substance, I began to gag. But instead of slowing down I picked up the pace, spitting all the way from Berm's Peak, down the backstretch, and into the Sungod Pool facilities, where I cleansed my palate at the water fountain next to the exercise room. *Oh, joy the sun* I thought as I exited the building, pulled the brim of my hat down and got back onto the track. Of course it had been out before, but always in a winter's air. On this cloudless day the sun's rays heated the air temperature to double digits on the Celsius scale, making it as tangible to run in as rain. It was a significant day in my training, as the seasonal change laid bare my complete and utter inexperience as a runner, with the pungent fingertip lick being only the first indication of what running in higher temperatures would have in store for me.

Oh boy, oh boy. After showering I sat on the couch and reflected on the session. I needed more water, less clothing, and a good dose of mental toughness to take on this most wicked of elements: ten degree Celsius heat stress.

It occurred to me that having a low finish time in the Sun Run would be the best way to combat this whole heat thing (you know, less time on the track equating to less time being exposed to the elements). I must have been waving my arms around, as I'm wont to do even when I'm talking to myself, and I got a whiff of a rancid smell that caused me to shudder with repulsion. I scanned the room looking for anyone—even Rosie—to accuse, but I was alone. I even looked out the window in some absurd attempt to lay the blame on someone walking on the street before I calmed down and got the nerve to smell myself. It was a touch-and-go operation because the small whiff that prompted the investigation provided just enough information to justify the possibility that I might upchuck when I came upon the source.

It took a minute or two. After checking out a few possible sources that produced minor nose wrinkling at just the thought of the regular smells, I came upon the irregular. It was my watch strap. The fuzzy Velcro-fastening system had soaked and stored all the sweat from previous weeks, and it was now emanating a cured and concentrated form of it as out-and-out stink. Although the taste, smell, and ensuing detox process of the strap in the bathroom sink were indelibly etched into my mind, they didn't make it to the hand-drawn lines of the log on that day. Instead, something much more positive was put into words when I scribbled that my right knee was not getting any worse.

Week 10

Session 1 44 minutes. Run 10 minutes, walk 1 minute.
Do this 4 times. Saturday, March 8, 2003.

Pre-dawn six days a week there is a loud thump against the cement foundation of the house followed by a long, smooth whoosh of a sound that starts and ends with a sharp clank of metal against metal. It's the *Vancouver Sun* newspaper being delivered through the mail slot with the consistency and dependability of an alarm clock. In fact, it *is* my alarm clock because it signals the beginning of my day. I may be up and at it with the delivery of the newspaper, but it would not be read until four hours later when I had come back from walking Emma to school. That is unless it was Monday, feature day for Sun Run training, in which case my need-to-know neurons would kick in and I would flop the paper down, then flip it open to section B and peruse the latest from Pete McMartin and reporter Jenny Lee.

My recent success, if the abatement of stink and an increase in my pain threshold can be categorized in this manner, had driven my desire to learn up a notch or two. The ban on Internet searches pertaining to well-being or exercise was still in effect (mostly to keep insurance premiums for self-surgery malpractice suits as low as possible). So this left me with two sources of learning: the original Document (and the exhaustive examination of its ongoing log) and the Monday morning *Vancouver Sun* newspaper.

I feel ashamed to admit to not having bought an armful of "how to run" books, but the bottom line was that I had more than enough information. By the time I took into account Shelly's and Nancy's experiences along with my own, then added a few layers of Jenny Lee articles, and of course threw in a dollop of Pete McMartin, I ended up with a multi-dimensional pot of knowledge from which to draw. You know, if I had kept the lawnmower jacket, the stopwatch, and the first pair of runners and just put up with sweat stinging my eyes instead of buying a high-tech hat, the whole initiative, including having access to the *Vancouver Sun*'s large breadth of knowledge, would have been considered cheap to boot.

Over the last couple of Mondays, Jenny Lee had given updates on the three runners-in-training that she was following. News anchor Steve Darling, an athletic man by any definition, had taken his training from the road to the track and then to the trails. I'm not talking about the gentle, undulating trails in an idyllic suburban park setting, like North Delta's McKitrick Park. I'm talking about the heavy-duty trails of the North Shore mountains. These are maintained trails, mind you, but they are rough and rugged, with a plethora of tripping hazards such as large stones and tree roots. There was no surface uniformity of asphalt covered with a layer of natural ground covering as in Vancouver's Stanley Park, or the rain-absorbing bark-mulch surface of the Sungod Track.

Steve seemed to be doing well, even having some fun, which was thought provoking in itself. At that point in time, smiling or even laughing while running would have caused me to lose the vital concentration required for putting one foot in front of the other. But I don't want to create a false impression, so in all honesty, even if I grimaced I still would not have had the mental acuity to run a mountain trail during week ten. Even so, it was encouraging to know that maybe some day I too could be laughing—you know, hyena-style—around the track.

Jenny Lee's update on stay-at-home mom Gwen was interesting because it dealt with a training activity that had been a constant source of scrutiny of mine since day one: stretching. Over the course of the first ten weeks, I had through trial and error adjusted my stretching to alleviate most of my tribulations. I had increased stretching on my left heel and stopped knee-bend stretching on my right knee. I was also reducing the right leg hamstring stretches during this period, which I thought was contributing to a happier, healthier knee.

The best part of the article was some commentary on doing a light jog, then doing some stretches. I didn't see this as an opportunity to eliminate stretching minutes, but by stretching closer to the track I could eliminate some other time-consuming things, such as scratching the dog. For Rosie it was automatic now that if I got down on the floor, she would come over and assume the position for her rightful scratches. In my ongoing quest to reduce the set-up time for my training sessions, I figured I would incorporate this jog and stop to stretch as opposed to stretch and stop to scratch, plus a few other organization-type ideas that I had come up with, into the coming sessions.

Morning radio host Erin Davis made me feel a touch uncomfortable as I read her training update. Erin, who learned to run in 2002 by following the Sun Run training program, recapped her post-run experience. In a nutshell, her personal fitness program fizzled big time after last year's run. Erin was now working on ways to make sure this did not happen again this year.

This is where the hair on the back of my neck stood up as I looked over my shoulder at the training Document on the fridge and read the statement written in red ink along the top. A hand-drawn arrow coming out of the end of the statement indicated the timeline. That timeline's conclusion was about a month away, and I had put zero thought into any follow-up routine. What I was doing was hard enough. I couldn't take the pressure of keeping up with Erin Davis's extended fitness outlook, nor could I compete with Steve Darling's gung-ho style, so I started in on the safe, comfortable territory of a Pete McMartin column.

McMartin opened up all his Sun Run columns with a revised statement of his goals. His goal during this week was to "sue my employer for physical and mental anguish." Goals from previous weeks included to "become so annoyingly fit my friends and family will come to resent me, more than they do now," and my favourite, "lose enough weight to do my own nude love scenes when the script calls for it." No doubt he would get Denny Boyd, who did a stint as a radio host who counselled callers' sex problems on a show called "Female Forum" during the seventies, to be the scriptwriter, thereby ensuring that said scenes would actually take place—and a scene I'm sure they would be.

Whether it was Jenny Lee or Pete McMartin, the coverage was motivational material that helped me get out the door, not just on Mondays but on all days of the week. There was only one problem, and that was the constant reference to the fact that I had to be registered. Oh, how I loathe having to commit. Wasn't worshipping the Document enough?

Session 2 41 minutes. Run 20 minutes, walk 1 minute, run 20 minutes. Monday, March 10, 2003.

"No, Dave, how many times do I have to tell you? I am not part of a secret society," said Shelly as we transitioned from running to walking. The exasperation and lilt of her voice coupled with a struggled intake of air made me turn towards her and size up the situation. Oh, it was a frightening sight as I saw crystal-clear droplets of sweat on my wife's brow for the first time in my life. Then the searing heat from the look that she flashed in my direction dried my own perspiration-soaked brow as she said, "And stop talking." This directive was followed up with my dry and military dictum, "We go again in three minutes."

Emma was at Brownies while we followed Shelly's training regime on the Sungod Track. In analyzing the Document, it turned out that all of week ten had reduced total training times, with this session having the least amount of time out on the track. I figured the spirit of the Document was to take it easy and give the body a break, so I chose to do just that and more by following Shelly's newbie regime on this day of training. This all sounds good in theory but it really was the perfect recipe for civil unrest not seen since the day the Hutchinsons couldn't figure out whether to run left or right around the park.

The countdown to running concluded, and in unison we picked up our pace, albeit in silence. Seconds later I could hear Shelly labouring with her breathing once more, and it was then that I realized I was passing the pregnancy test with flying colours. Of course I wasn't pregnant, but according to one of Jenny Lee's articles my heart rate was in the proper zone. The safe heart rate criteria for pregnant women could be measured in their ability to carry on a conversation while running. Up to that run repetition, I had been talking up a storm, firstly because I could; having someone to actually talk to was a distant second. Most of the gabbing was because my wife had infused in me an insatiable need for clarification of an earlier comment that had resonated through my grey matter file directories with unsatisfactory results.

We had just hit the track, and I was in a full dogmatic tutorial on how Shelly should put one foot in front of the other when she said, "Dave, I'm not in CGIT anymore." I was stunned, and not because her inflection indicated that she had had her fill of my expository nature— we had long ago attained consensus that I was an overpiped bag of Celtic wind. No, I was stunned because I didn't know the meaning of CGIT.

The problem with people who think they've heard it all is that when something does come along that they haven't heard about, they think it must be somehow unique and special. So as I jaunted along the track while Shelly pushed, dragged, and plodded, I did my best imitation of Pete McMartin and questioned her on what in the world CGIT was. Filling out the acronym of Canadian Girls In Training was the easy part; getting the details was a different story.

I guess all the evasive non-answers I received that day from my partner of more than ten years put me on a secrecy tack that seemed a perfect fit to a question I'd had about our relationship from day one. Specifically, why did I have to ask Shelly to marry me so many times? I have to tell you that at the time it was as close to begging as any man wants to admit to, but in the dim light of that day's training it all made sense. Oh sure, if I was being brought into a secret society and all there would need to be some sort of period of time—where paperwork, handshakes, or whatever got approved. This would explain all the no's.

I was feeling mighty pleased with the secret society theory, then Shelly cemented the angle by saying that Trudy had also been in CGIT. I stumbled upon hearing this. I couldn't believe it. Trudy and Mel, our neighbours? Like Shelly, Trudy had grown up in Vancouver's West End, where she had received her training as well. It was shortly after finding out about Trudy that I was told to stop talking about it, which enabled me to live the secret society fantasy until I met Trudy out on the lawn the next day. She burst my bubble with the revelation that CGIT was a version of Brownies/Girl Guides. Hey, I didn't have any idea. Not a clue.

We ended the run/walk session on the south side behind the Sungod Pool when Shelly just couldn't take it anymore (the running or me), so just after a small group of ivy-entrenched alder trees, she took the low road, leaving me to handle the high road. During construction of the pool extension, a new trail was created that went around both the construction zone and the berm created from the original pool construction. With a minute left in the session, Shelly took the flat detour while I danced and pranced up then down the grade, where I waited for her to emerge from behind a long row of ten-foot-tall cedar trees at the end of the detour path. It truly was a display unbecoming of a gentleman.

Oh, did I get an earful on the walk home. I may have stopped talking to Shelly, but the reduced heart rate of the session had me in an exuberant mood, where I talked to everybody else we came in contact with. You know, the lifeguard on a break, some boys playing ball hockey in the parking lot, dog walkers, not to mention a quick hi to other joggers as they passed us.

"Who do you think you are, do-gooder Mr. Rogers, and isn't it a wonderful day in the neighbourhood? It's like I'm the one who married into some society: the Odd Fellows, with you being a full-fledged member," said Shelly with a huff and a puff and a profane expletive between every third word.

You would have thought I had mocked her. You know with my hands over my mouth, doing a PNE-style carnival ride operator voice in complete public-address-speaker blown distortion and yelling, "Do you want to go faster?" Of course I hadn't, but I had taken a measure of pleasure in the fact that her training was going to have some sort of difficulty factor attached to it, because the suddenness and then the ease with which she had started her training had unnerved me.

As it turned out, this was the last time during my Sun Run training that Shelly trained with me. I guess we are more alike than not, and once she figured out that there was going to be some pain involved in learning to run, she preferred to handle it solo. Another factor in Shelly's running solo was the daily sunset times, which were getting closer to seven o'clock, enabling her to get home from work and run in the daylight. This was also Shelly's last time on the Sungod Track; she took her routine to the streets in a display of intrepid behaviour that did more to give me pause than any cantankerous request for silence ever did.

Session 3 45 minutes. Run 22 minutes, walk 1 minute, run 22 minutes. Thursday, March 13, 2003.

Mirrors? I don't need to show myself to any stinking mirrors. Well, except for shaving, if only to avoid rounding off all my facial high points and becoming a zero (you know, the one before the one). Like bathroom scales, the mirror and any of its reflective cousins are a source of dread and anguish. I say this just so you know how unusual it was for me to be standing fully clothed in front of the bathroom mirror, with one hand wiping the fogged mirror while the other hand lifted my shirt.

I had finished the third run in week ten and written, "Did it again," in the log, taken a shower, then startled myself while getting dressed. It was a hand travelling too far that got my attention as I realized I had reclaimed another notch in my belt. I repeated the process a few more times to determine if the notch was the result of a good cinch gone wrong or even if I was suffering from some sort of exercise-induced spatial breakdown where I had actually lost a notch, the accepted norm for many years.

As I peered into the fog-shrouded mirror, the visual determination of weight loss all seemed so ambiguous—until I saw my ribs. I rubbed the mirror harder and was lifting my shirt higher in order to ward off any potential shadows when, holy wishbone, it became apparent that it indeed was a ridgeline of ribs that I was witnessing for the first time this millennium. My torso had definition; it wasn't a blotched, over-ripe pear with a mottle of grey and black hair anymore. I whipped off my shirt and wiped the mirror with bigger swirls in anticipation of additional weight loss. I stood back and checked out my stomach, and when I was unsatisfied with the results I leaned forward and wiped the mirror again. When there was no change, I bent over and checked the notch on my belt. Oh, I hadn't lost the reclaimed notch, but the stomach looked as soft and rotund as ever.

Now I must admit that this was the second notch I had reclaimed, but the first notch didn't have much credibility because it was a Christmas notch. At Christmas, with all the shortcake, chocolate, and boatloads of gravy, I had gained a notch, which by the way was the last notch on my belt. Of course, coming to the end of the line on my belt did not mean that weight loss was a reason for starting up this whole training initiative (you know, to avoid retooling the wardrobe). I've said it before and I'll say it again—weight loss was not a training objective. Anyway, I reclaimed that notch in the first week of training and wrote it off as the instrument calibration process.

I wiped a little higher in order to see the ridgeline of ribs again, then noticed that my neck appeared to be thinned out. This was where the hardcore evidence of weight loss could be seen and not merely measured. My neck, shoulders, and the tops of my arms looked positively skinny, but instead of feeling good about this, some type of Poh-Poh course of thought prevailed and I had to turn my back on the mirror on the wall and leave the bathroom.

I sat perched on the edge of the wingback chair, ready to take some yet-to-be-determined course of action against the onslaught of ill health, because seeing that skinniness and all didn't make me feel good, not one iota. Even with the elevated heart rate due to the recently completed training run to remind me of the reason for the weight loss, I could not escape the deleterious thoughts of impending doom.

I got through the rest of the day by keeping myself busy, first by taking the dog for a walk. It was a reflex action to get outside again and clear my head, but it didn't escape my attention that I was doing more of this exercise thing, which was possibly masking a serious health condition. Later that day I still wasn't doing much better, and when I looked in the mirror again and saw the ridgeline of ribs, I thought it looked like a big frown. A hairy one at that but still a frown, reminding me that I should be vigilant and continue to be on the lookout for other ill-fated health signs.

Meanwhile, the Vancouver Sun Run was exactly one month away from this day, yet I had no interest in registering. What was the point if I was going to be too diseased to participate? I suppose I should have known better, and anyone I know would have said I should have known better. And I suppose I should have been happy, and anyone I know would have said, "Dave, be happy." But I didn't and I couldn't and I wasn't about to.

Week 11

It was early Saturday morning and I'd found a comfort zone while reading the 1941 Governor General's Literary Award–winner for general literature, Klee Wyck, when I heard a slow, rhythmic thump of heavy footsteps coming down the stairs. Instinctively I exchanged the Emily Carr memoir for the *Sun* newspaper. The *Sun* was bigger, heavier, and had removable sections, so it could be considered a superior multi-purpose tool compared with the format of the memoir. If approached by a friend, I could use the paper to make myself look potentially useful by being able to answer questions about tide tables and whatnot, and if approached by a foe, I could use it as a swatting tool. Then there was the old stand-by newspaper use of draping it over oneself while sleeping on a park bench in order to keep warm should the footsteps turn out to be a harbinger of being tossed from the house.

When I heard the guttural muttering accompanying the footsteps, it was as if I had been subjected to an unfortunate eighties flashback that jolted me out of my chair, rendering both the book and newspaper ineffectual as they fell about the kitchen floor. Shelly rounded the corner with her hair tossed and matted, her untied housecoat hanging precariously on her slim shoulders like a picked-over garment on a Bay Day rack. One hand reached out in a purpose-driven manner for the coffee, stale as it was. Oh, and the muttering never stopped.

In an attempt to thwart the horror of the moment I turned on the radio, hoping to hear the soothing, world-is-at-peace sounds of a Michael Buble track. The punk rock lyrics by the band D.O.A. that were spewing from my wife were the result of her being subjected to a fir-tree splitting, headboard-vibrating musical onslaught over the course of her sleep from the neighbours' teenagers' party the night before.

Of course Shelly was mocking the late-night rattle-and-hum event, as she actually detested everything from the choice of music, the volume, and the timing of it all. As for me, well, I kind of liked it.

From my first audio experience years ago, I was blown away by the neighbours' stereo's ability to attain loud and proud volume levels. It wasn't a question of room acoustics or transistors versus tubes, and it wasn't a matter of high end versus low end or flat-out bulging bags of money. What it all came down to was synergy. The boys were able to attain beastly levels of volume by using components that worked well with each other, in this case exceedingly well.

After doing the pillow-propped double-blind test, not seeing or knowing what components were in use, I was hard pressed to say if one component was superior to another. Each component got an above-average rating, but none of them came close to achieving a check mark in the outstanding category. For instance, the amp sure had the juice, but it got its mark for what it didn't do: cry under the voltage strain of playing raw heavy metal tunes. The speakers must have had some surface area to them, and I rarely heard them falter, but they were missing the muscular slam needed for a higher mark. The CD player was the most intriguing of all since it provided a surprising open and unrestricted feel to the music.

Of course the open and newly green expanse of my backyard provided the perfect conduit for the tuneful version of the Guess Who's

"Share the Land." The overall effect of these middle-of-the-road components was a classic case of the whole being bigger, better, and of course a-whole-lotta-love louder than any of its individual parts. Now, I've cued this particular stereo story because between it and Shelly, I came to view the Sungod Track differently. Over coffee that morning, she had been telling me about her last two solo runs, which were done on cement (that is, the sidewalk), when in mid-sentence she took a sip of coffee and then gestured in a graceful manner across the table with a soft and dainty open hand, the inference being, *Like hey, big boy, what's your biggest problem?* This struck so hard she might as well have leaned a little further over the table and grabbed a fistful of chest hair, then yelled longshoreman style into my face.

It was then and there that I realized that leaving the Sungod Track wasn't something that fell into the nice-to-do category of getting in a couple of concrete runs before the big event. It was now in the must-do category, if for no other reason than to develop some running synergy if I was going to attain my training objectives. Well, okay, I guess keeping up to both Shelly and Nancy had something to do with it as well. I had to go beyond babying myself against shin splints or shielding myself against torn cartilage. I needed to learn from the teen sonica next door and form a synergy with a hard running surface or else this singular weak link could be the ruin of my Sun Run 2003 experience.

After coffee with Shelly, I went for my training run and soft-pedalled around the immediate neighbourhood for twenty-one minutes before heading out to the Sungod Track. To counterbalance my apprehension of incurring an injury on the hard running surface, I put myself through a refresher course of what I had learned about running to date, with a focus on a biomechanically correct form (chin up, arms relaxed, and feet landing properly with each step).

Now it may appear that I was being smart by running only twenty-one minutes in the neighbourhood and gradually building up to running full time on hard surfaces, but why would intelligence suddenly become a factor in my training? It was only twenty-one minutes because the refresher course was cost free, and that included any cost to my dignity. You see, I was still having trouble with the whole walking aspect of this training initiative, and I wanted to make sure I was well within the comforting confines of the Sungod Track when the walk portion of this session started at the twenty-five minute mark.

The familiarity of the track on the soles of my mesh-panelled babies was heaven sent, and because I had held back early in the session on the road, my breathing was far from being laboured. The resulting euphoria that took hold set the scenario for the evaluation portion of my refresher course. On the south-side berm behind the Sungod Pool, the then newly installed timer board was on (some days during this installation period it was powered down). With my watch set to count the Document's prescribed training time, I used the pool timer board to time each lap around the track. I suppose I could have dual-tasked my watch, but I'm sure the inordinate amount of time spent looking at my wrist would have increased the risk of serious injury from running into the trunk of some obstinate tree.

Now I'd used the timer board to monitor the speed aspect of my performance in the past, so I knew I had set a personal best when on each of the last two laps my time just squeezed under the nine-minute mark. There was elation, but it wasn't displayed with fist-pumping hands over the head. Instead, it was hands on the knees while I vacuumed a section of the track just out of view of most pool patrons—the exception being a lifeguard who had stepped up to the window and placed one leg on the ledge as he watched me. I truly hoped this was a humanitarian gesture on his behalf and that he was at the ready to dust off his life-saving skills should I have inhaled and then choked on a piece of bark mulch. Well, the Heimlich manoeuvre wasn't required, and because of this I guess I could categorize the first session of week eleven, which also included my first strides off the track, as a success.

WEEK 11

Session 2 56 minutes. Run 30 minutes, walk 1 minute, run 25 minutes. Tuesday, March 18, 2003.

You'd think I would have had enough of the track after running it three times a week for ten full weeks, but not really, not even by a long shot. You'd think I would have seen everything there was to see, but not really. Magnolia trees were blooming in some of the private yards that back onto the park, hardly making for stale, ho-hum viewing. You'd think that loneliness and despair would have gotten the best of me, but I was far from alone. My Tiny Tim tiptoeing had progressed to a lope around the loop, where I frequently saw Goldy and Sandy, two lab/cocker crosses, out on their daily walk with mama Myrtle, whose word was always obeyed. Then there were Cody and Isabella, a pair of bichon/shih tzu crosses who were visitors to the park whenever their grandmother was looking after them. Plus, how could you be lonely when there was competition at hand? I'd made a friend in the park that I named Norway. Norway was a fat, bushy-tailed black squirrel who liked to run with me. The little plumper perched on top of the fence along the south end of the track and stared me down until I was even with him, then he raced forward about twenty feet. He'd focus one beady eye on me again until I'd caught up to him, then he regained the lead. Norway hadn't lost a race all season.

Of course, I came across more than just animals out on the track. There were the teenagers who liked to smooch where the ice shavings were piled from the hockey rink; biology had most likely determined this location. There was the older eastern European speed walker who zipped in the opposite direction to me, for which I was eternally thankful. The pair of three-ton boulders by the track's backstretch generated a magnetic pull that attracted only customer service representative vehicles. Maybe the secluded parking spot was scheduled and that was what the consistent rotation of cars was

201

all about—their occupants talking on their phones, booking and rebooking the spaces.

The parking lot where I normally entered the park off of 112th Street usually had mothers sitting in vans waiting for their children's swim classes to end, and the parking lot by Berm's Peak filled up only in the evenings when there was a junior hockey game taking place. This open space during the day was used by people learning how to in-line skate or how to park a car. Don't worry, these have never been simultaneous activities, although I remember hopping in a cab in Winnipeg one winter's night many years ago and finding the driver wearing ice skates. You know, I never got around to asking him about the skates because I was too busy asking about the stack of pizzas he was delivering.

You'd think I would have had enough of McKitrick Park and the Sungod Track, but no, there I was walking Rosie on it after using it for that day's training session. I chose not to run on cement for this session because my right knee was feeling a bit strange (the mashed-potato syndrome was making a comeback after running off-track for the first time).

I was lost in thought as I walked along the track and looked across the street through the floor-to-ceiling windows in the newly created exercise room. I was taking note of the standardized gait of the runners on the treadmill machines when I felt the ground pound. I knew that Rosie felt it too because she stopped walking, looked back over her shoulder, then put her tail between her legs and leaned in tight against my shin, forcing me to stop walking too. I then heard the sound of thunder, and my skin sensed an air pressure change that was accompanied by the sight of the back of a young male's sweaty T-shirt. Then another and another and another appeared before our eyes.

Within seconds, at least twenty T-shirts had passed us, then they made an abrupt stop at the foot of Berm's Peak, where an older male stood hunched over a stopwatch. It didn't take long before Rosie and I were in the middle of the huffing and puffing group of runners as they milled about the finish line. I asked the timer who they were, and he told me this was his grade-eight class from Burnsview. Burnsview School is located a block and a half away from the Sungod Track on 112th Street.

I picked up Rosie and sought out the winner of the race by wading into a tighter-packed group of boys off to the side. The winner was a strapping young lad who was taller than I was and had big clodhoppers that were disproportional to his height. Now I don't really know what a runner's high is, but I don't believe I was walking around under its influence, and of course I don't do mind-expanding drugs, but the whole class seemed to have big feet. That's why I picked up the little white dog.

The winner was in a jovial mood with his pals when I walked up and asked him for his finish time. This produced a mega-watt smile that accentuated his leading-man good looks, worthy of any Harlequin paperback cover. I almost dropped the dog when he told me a time of three minutes and forty-one seconds. I shuffled off up Berm's Peak, stunned at the thought of a speed that was close to three times faster than my personal best around the track. Oh, such glory, to truly be a rocketman, to stretch ligaments where no ligaments have been stretched before.

The whole pain aspect brought me to my senses, and I reverted back to the analytical side of things, like wondering if I too created a vacuum when I passed somebody. This produced a chortle that got lost in the clear air of the fifteen-foot-high Berm's Peak. Pass somebody? Me? I was still wary of being passed by any walker within eyeball range. I wasn't about to mess up someone else's hair with a rubber-sole-generated maelstrom.

At the end of the walk I bent over to unleash the dog, then rubbed my knee before straightening up. As much as I liked the Sungod Track, I knew I had to take my show on the road.

Session 3   51 minutes. Run 40 minutes, walk 1 minute,
run 10 minutes. Thursday, March 20, 2003.

First it was a mother pushing a baby carriage, then it was the eastern
European speed walker, now it was the postman. Yes, the dude who
delivers the mail. What can I say? The competition was wide, varied,
and completely unexpected.

This was my first full training session off of the Sungod Track,
and I thought I would warm up to the task by doing a quick lap around
the block. Well, okay, once again I was proving to myself that I could
dawdle with the best of them. I got about halfway around when I got
a feeling way down deep at the bottom of my fresh white socks that
I was good to go.

I released some tension with a Toller Cranston hand roll, then
executed a rare right turn and found myself out in the cacophony of
traffic and life in general on 80th Avenue. Gone were the predictable
patterns of conservative and pretty much static greens and browns,
and my eyes darted one way then another as I chased down all the
swirling colours they were replaced with. I fumbled with my hat and
watch, then checked the key holder on my shoe as I made a frantic
attempt to calm myself with something familiar and comforting . . .
and then it happened.

A flash of deep, dark blue on blue emerged from a driveway and
matched my step stride for stride. It was Russ the running postman,
with a bag over each shoulder, delivering the mail. Oh, I had seen Russ
and his unique method of getting the job done before, but always at a
distance while I walked Emma to school on the other side of the street
or while I was driving by in the car. In my most perspiration-soaked
Chariots of Fire dreams, I had never gone shoulder to shoulder with
the postman, and this lack of visualization was the likely source of the
tightness that started in my chest and inched its way up to my throat.

A few strides later and my arms ached as if I were carrying his bags, albeit bellhop style.

I had just thrown my head back and was about to quit and start walking when he gave me a wave of the wrist reminiscent of a Kurt Browning championship performance and started down the next driveway. The release from competition brought instant relief, and the mesh-panelled babies never did stop. In fact, a few moments later I took a peek over my shoulder and was surprised by how much distance they had put between me and the postman.

That was the closest I came to not completing one of the Document's training sessions. Oh, it would have been easy to let go of my immediate objective of just getting to 112th Street, but before I knew it I had made another rare right turn at the mental goalpost and left my crushing encounter with the postman even farther behind.

The route I had picked followed the north end of 112th Street starting from 80th Avenue, because after eleven weeks of harassing Nancy about where the flattest routes were and then driving them, I figured this was it. Minutes into my northward journey I began to wonder about myself. Like why was I going so fast? I did a form and posture checklist, then checked the watch. Every aspect was in the *excellent* range. I found it astonishing how I could bounce back from the lowest of lows and hit an unprecedented high.

It took a few more minutes but I finally figured out at least one of the reasons, and that was the shoes. This was the first time I had run in them on a hard surface after being warmed up. As good as the Sungod Track was, its very nature of being a soft track went hand in hand with being a slow track. I figured I was feeling the real potential of the mesh-panelled babies for the first time as they seemed to assist my progress down the street.

The integration of foot and shoe had a mechanical feel to it, definitely a new experience, unnatural at that. I felt a sense of cheating as the mesh-panelled babies propelled my bulk up and over curbs then through the intersections they enclosed. After the 84th Avenue intersection, my fingers went from potato-chip-carrying mode to full poke-the-air extension as I picked up the pace and attained speed normally associated with golden figments of my imagination.

In *The Stone Diaries*, Cuyler Goodwill travels outside the province of Manitoba for the first time in his life. The journey represents the start of the quarryman's becoming a champion of commerce, the second major change that the character undertakes during the novel. There is nothing like a character changing his mannerisms, altering his outlook on life, or flat-out finding religion to stoke a reader's interest. One reason Cuyler is able to make these changes is because he was a student of people and the world around him. As he travelled by rail between Manitoba and Indiana, an aspect that caught his fancy was the flat prairie and its vast expanse. Cuyler was taken aback as he watched other travellers' nonchalant and seemingly disrespectful response to covering great distances.

I don't know what physical clues Cuyler looked for in these people in order to make his assessment of them, but it's possible he was looking for the same fear I believe he himself possessed on that trip. If this was the case, then he would have recognized the expression on my face when I competed the "out" portion of the training session and turned at Annieville Park to head back home. It was all uphill, which was so unexpected.

As it turned out, I had been running down a very slight grade. No wonder it had felt so good. I started by digging in and fixing my eyes on the top of the grade. After repeating to myself *It looks so far away* about ten times over, my fear was overtaken by anger, which was quickly replaced with anxiety as I couldn't stop looking at the watch. This was no Berm's Peak, where the pain of the grade lasted but a few minutes; the duration of this pain looked to be infinite, which made wishing for the one-minute walk more like a desperate beg. My emotions sure were scrambled at the beginning of the return portion of this training session, but strangely ten minutes later when the walk portion came due, I had to actually force myself to walk. The

Document had come through again, as it had me more than prepared for this physical challenge. All I needed to do was believe in it.

As I reflected on the session, I had to admit there were some flaws in my training preparedness on this day, starting with my lack of gumption in dealing with the postman's challenge and ending with my fear of inclines. After poring over this aspect of my training in the Document, I found much to my chagrin that it didn't address this low gumption quotient.

In an attempt to soothe all that ailed me, I fired up the tubes and threw on the progressive piano harmonies of a Renee Rosnes CD. I sucked on an orange slice and mulled over the dilemma of not only being soft physically but possibly being even softer mentally. You see, it had taken years to attain such a low gumption quotient rating, and making changes in this department before the Sun Run was going to be difficult if not impossible since I had no idea how. Where was the accompanying Sun Run training psychological development Document?

Week 12

66 minutes. Run 45 minutes, walk 1 minute, run 20 minutes. Saturday, March 22, 2003.

I just didn't have the time to reset the trip odometer, drive a bit, turn right then right some more, then get out and survey the land from a runner's perspective. This quest for flatness was a time-consuming process, and the returns were anything but guaranteed as my last run proved. Plus I was beginning to feel uneasy about driving around the neighbourhood so often. Years ago I remember seeing an American television news feature where a high-level CIA operative was accused of being a double agent, partly on the basis of having a suspicious-looking map in his possession. The map turned out to be a plan for a future running route. Now I'm pretty sure that CSIS, Canada's spy agency, wasn't watching me, but maybe granny sitting in the front window figured I was casing her street.

So time and paranoia put me back in the park, which was probably a good thing since the inside of my right knee felt as if it had just been hit with a frozen hockey puck. Hard to believe, but I considered this an acceptable feeling if only because of its familiarity from some distant ice age and the tag-along knowledge that the pain was short term and not debilitating. The problem with this rationale was I had no recollection of any recent blunt trauma—well, at least to the body area in question—which left only wishful thinking on my behalf. Although this wishful thinking was how I got myself out the door in this first session of week twelve, I hope you can see how it wasn't strong enough reasoning to lay down cold cash to register for the Sun Run.

All motivational thoughts of Pete McMartin or Jenny Lee articles were heaped to one side for this training session because the reviews were in. It had been a regular firestorm of emotions that week as phone calls and face-to-face meetings resulted in a full spectrum of reviews for my cousin Ross Laird's book. I can't really say why this week of all weeks things came to a head, but his book, *Grain of Truth*, had received national attention the month before Christmas when it was short-listed for the 2002 Governor General's Literary Award. Although the book failed to win, the award ceremony explained all the hoopla. As far as the time lapse goes, I suspect it says more about me and how I've grown used to the high-tech world and my expectations of high-speed information gathering and dissemination. But book reading operates in a different, slower realm, and it was my folly to expect anything else.

Now let me attest to the fact that the older style of communication makes up for its lack of speed by letting things simmer a bit longer, which exponentially increases the seething factor. *Grain of Truth* explores woodworking in a contemplative and spiritual manner, but it was the family aspect of the memoir that most of its critics took exception to. To succinctly put it, the public airing of his mother's drunkenness went over as well as a long-stemmed glass of red wine on a white carpet. There was a degree of elegance in the initial tipping stage because people were pleased with his award nomination, but the resulting permeation in the final stage of spilling cast a dark stain that would be difficult if not impossible to undo.

I was close to Ross's mother (my dad's sister) and loved her very much. I had trouble myself reading about her, but there is no denying that she drank excessive amounts of alcohol. By the end of her life, she had formed battlefronts with her husband, with Ross, and with her brother, the latter placing me in the collateral damage category.

Once Granddad and I are added into the mix, I have had a first-person account of an alcohol-fuelled generational madness that has ripped through a century of time and across two continents. Ground zero to the best of my knowledge was Red Hill, County Caven, Northern Ireland. It won't make any itinerary of mine.

While I completed my run on the Sungod Track, with all laps under the nine-minute mark, I considered a second point in the reviews, which had garnered a universal response of "He sure can write." Man alive, can he ever. He had penned more than one description of woodworking tools, particularly the knives, that I could only marvel at—I was way past envy.

Session 2 66 minutes. Run 50 minutes, walk 1 minute, run 15 minutes. Tuesday, March 25, 2003.

I'd like to point out that although cousin Ross's memoir *Grain of Truth* was number one during all fireside chats in this period, I never once gave any thought to writing a memoir, let alone a memoir that had a running theme. I had other things on my mind, such as why didn't I feel like a runner?

After much soul searching I came up with the remedy to this whole business of not feeling like a runner—while walking home, of all things, after taking Emma to school. The answer to addressing my low gumption quotient lay in the Document after all, which pleased me to no end. If there were grannies out there watching my every move on their streets, they would have been asking themselves, "Who's that grinning fool?" since the more I thought about it, the bigger my smile got. I stormed the back door, donned my running gear, and threw myself into a set of warm-up exercises. When I finished the first set, I did another and then another. After the third set I hammered my way up the flight of stairs, turned, and took a breath.

It was just like the old days—you know, the start of all this training a mere twelve weeks ago. With sweat streaming down my face, I took a few deep breaths in preparation of chasing away all my insecurities about being a runner. You see, I was about to go for it because the Document told me so. Or at least that was my interpretation as I continued to stand at the top of the stairs with the lights off.

In my assessment of that day's training session, I had determined that it was the apex of the endurance aspect of the Document; no other session would have as much running time on the track. There were three more sessions after this one, but they all had reduced training times. I guess it would be like gearing down before the big day.

I figured there was no better way to overcome the pervasive negative anticipation I had for my participation in the Sun Run 2003 than by actually proving to myself that I could go the distance. So this was it, show time, where I decided to put it all on the line. I was going to take advantage of the spirit of the Document and overshoot its stated length of time by running ten kilometres. With the absence of any mental noise, I visualized each of the planned ten laps on the Sungod Track, and when my heart rate had sufficiently calmed, I knew I was good to go.

I made my way down the stairs, out the back door, down the driveway, and round the willow tree. I turned at Audrey and Ted's, and then, just like my meeting with the running postman, my weakest muscle was put to the test.

Confusion rained down hard as I tried to make sense of what was before me. Cars, cars, and more cars were parked up and down the entire street, including the side streets. Although I was more than a bit troubled by it all, I made things worse by wondering if Poh-Poh would have interpreted the walling of the street with sheet metal as a sign for all marauding runners to stay clear of the park.

I'd never seen so many cars in the neighbourhood. I'd never even heard of this many cars being in the neighbourhood. My pace slowed considerably as I surveyed the landscape and tried to formulate a plausible answer.

When I reached 112th Street the situation was even worse: cars were parked in every available space in both north and south directions. I entered the trail to the Sungod Track and could see through the trees that the parking lot next to the swimming pool was full as well. This gave me my first clue as to what in the world was going on. Obviously there was a special event of some sort at the recreation centre, but what? My eyes scanned the Delta Parks and Recreation reader board to no avail, but as I turned up the entranceway boulevard, it all became quite clear. The solid gloss-white sides of trailers on one side of the ice rink's parking lot were indisputable evidence of the movie industry in full mobilization.

As I made my way across the crosswalk at the foot of Berm's Peak, a security guard gave me a friendly wave and a cheerful smile. I gave her a quick wave back, but my attention quickly returned to the track because industry types were crossing it in a leisurely fashion, and I didn't want to get tripped up. The resulting strain of doing a zigzag on and off the track caused my chest to tighten during the ascent of Berm's Peak. Once at the peak, I swallowed hard and looked down on the tents and the food trucks at that end of the parking lot. It was a mumbo-jumbo scene of people, trucks, trailers, and tents that put me totally off my game, forcing me to begin the process of reconsidering that day's objective.

It felt strange to be choked up with stress, disillusioned about having my big day messed with, and fascinated by my surroundings all at the same time. Down the backstretch and behind the pool I tried to make the decision of going home or going on, then the one-kilometre data came in at the end of the first lap as I pressed the lap counter on my watch. Oh, baby, seven and a half minutes. A smokin' world record as far as I was concerned—no wonder I was having trouble breathing. With the quantitative data in hand I made the decision to continue, but I slowed my pace in an attempt to stave off suffocation and give myself reasonable odds at completion.

The security guard at the foot of Berm's Peak gave me a thumbs-up on the second lap, and by the time I was on the fourth lap she was giving me a round of applause. I'm not one to go out of my way to bring attention to myself, and strange as it may sound the clapping didn't prompt one extra eyeball to scrutinize my form. The reason for that was they were all on me already. It was as if the unit production manager had brought me in to entertain the masses. From the food lineups, to the generator areas, to the zone surrounding the gleaming trailers people were watching the man in red go round and round the park. It was all a little embarrassing.

The beginning of lap eight was the start of venturing into total training times and distances that were beyond anything I had trained for up to that point, so in a planned move I deviated off the track for a sip of water inside the recreation centre. During this water break I saw that the movie shoot was taking place inside the ice rink. As I hustled out, the security guard met me at the doors, giving my stomach that churning feeling one gets before receiving a traffic ticket. She then held out her hand, which to my relief didn't have a writing pad or a pair of cuffs in it, and in a chipper voice said, "The Marathon Man." It took another moment, but I finally figured out that she wanted me to give her a high-five. Well that was pretty nice and all, but where was the crowd control? I was not used to strange women smiling at me and wanting to touch, so I ran away.

It occurred to me somewhere on lap nine that maybe she was making reference to the 1976 movie *Marathon Man* and that maybe she wanted my autograph. Lap ten finished with me thinking about going back and signing her vest. I can now look back and say that my first excursion into long-distance running had debilitated my thought processes in a serious manner.

Session 3 45 minutes. Run 45 minutes. Friday, March 28, 2003.

The last three laps of my 10K test run may have enfeebled my mind, but after seeing my shirt hanging loosely about my gut after the run I figured it was worth it. Oh, I know I said this whole running initiative wasn't about weight loss, but the lack of protuberance from the middle of my untucked shirt got me excited enough to put a rare exclamation point in the Document's comments section.

I really should have been thinking about how I had overcome the psychological barriers of running 10K and completing a run without walking, but all I could think of was cousin Helen and her scale. Yes, how much did I weigh? While drying the dishes later that night, I spoke to Shelly about the test run and scheduling a weigh-in at cousin Helen's. I was getting the appropriate ahhs and yesses, which fuelled my confabulation, when a comment of "Not with me" brought my tale to an abrupt end. It seems I had started talking about running with my shirt off, and Shelly was drawing a line in the soapsuds on anything of the sort. Oh, I wasn't happy about the terse comment, which I saw as a negation of all I had accomplished that day, so I immediately went into negotiation mode.

I think we were discussing a blue moon somewhere in the Yukon in a very frozen and distant future when a crushing demand entered the stainless sink arena of debate. I had to shave my back. Oh, I ended the negotiations right there as I wagged a finger and told her I wasn't about to let reality TV, which was really fiction, get in the way of my reality. Of course I got the strangest look. There was no doubt that the new-fangled reality shows with skinny young guys shaving themselves on deserted islands and all were putting a lot of pressure on guys like me. In the end, though, having to keep my shirt on was just as well because I wasn't all that skinny; it was just a matter of the peak being pounded down after hours and hours of running, that's all. Density now made up for whatever depth I had once possessed.

Now, I had scoped out a concrete route that was meticulously measured, from the willow tree out through a predicted epic workout and back to the willow tree, but I didn't have the confidence to try it on this day of training because I was too tired. The 10K test at eighty-eight minutes had drained me, so I drove down to a Burns Bog trail that started near the Alex Fraser Bridge and did this session's forty-five-minute run there. The family had walked this flat route many times over the years, so I was familiar with it. The trail also had mixed surfaces of packed dirt, gravel, and asphalt, which fit my need of introducing myself to the harder surfaces that would be used in the Sun Run.

At the beginning of the session I took a little side route and ran up some stairs that brought me to Nordel Way, a steep causeway to the Alex Fraser Bridge. I took a look eastward and made a mental note of the grade for future reference. Could it be a possible running route? Maybe, but it would be a major feat based on the fact that I'd only ever seen two people running up it.

I made my way down the stairs and started a slow, purposeful run along the flat trail while I filled my mind with a review of the 10K test. A few things became apparent during that Marathon Man run, such as my lack of experience.

Although I had a planned water break, I think I came close to heat exhaustion because I was overclothed. The jacket had been great in its versatility, with its zippers and Velcro and all, but the weather was getting warmer and it was raining less every time out, which put the jacket's continued use into question. It could be rolled into a pouch and fastened around my waist, but my first attempt in the living room on a non-running day had not been all that successful, so I didn't attempt it out on the track. The long cotton pants I wore had been a problem as well. They had felt as hot and heavy as woolen trousers would have in 1940, the year that Poh-Poh died. I replayed what Poh-Poh would have said, "You only need to pay attention." I took Poh-Poh's commentary to heart along with the fact that I had been thinking about the era in which she died and believed during the run that the pants had become a sign that my past history was about to weigh me down.

So, the clothing aspect had certainly been a major problem, and that was before the sun even came out. The sun had become a tangible part of that session, making me think I was plodding my way through depression era dustbowl conditions—no wonder I became delirious. There had been very few sunny training days, so I was not used to running under the sun regardless of the air temperature, which was probably around ten degrees Celsius that day. I was wearing the exact clothes for the run on the bog trail two days later and was comfortable, which only added to my problem of not knowing what to do. The clothing issue and my general lack of experience was now my number one concern, even overriding my deep-seated fear of injury, which had slipped from a three-alarm, all-hands-on-deck crisis to whining air-raid-siren status.

The second thing that became apparent during the 10K Marathon Man run was that I just wasn't battle tested against other runner's. My comfort zone while running was so restricted that having someone wave at me threw me off my game plan. I remember running backwards for a few steps on the Burns Bog trail while reviewing this aspect of my performance, and after seeing absolutely no other runner's I had no choice but to give myself a failing grade.

So, my clothing and being battle tested were big-time issues that I worked on while running for the first time on a route without an incline. By the end of the forty-five-minute run I had a corrective action plan in place: it was time to shed some gear and enter a race.

Week 13

Session 1   50 minutes. Run 50 minutes. Sunday, March 30, 2003.

Nancy the powerbabe from down the street always countered my question of where she ran with "Did you sign up for the Run for Life yet?" Of course I hadn't. If I hadn't signed up for the Sun Run, why would I have signed up for some lesser local run? Well, that was my thinking up until the Burns Bog run, when I decided that the 5K community run in which all proceeds went to the Canadian Cancer Society was the perfect supplement to my Sun Run training.

The Run for Life was going to be a road race, which fit my hard-surfaces training criteria. I had no idea what streets the route took, which left me wanting, but at least it started in the familiar territory of McKitrick Park, home of the Sungod Track. The run would complement the Document's regimen by having me train against other participants. I didn't have a clue how many, which again was a cause for concern, but if I was to toughen up in this area I had to show up and take on the masses. Honestly, at this point I spent about 50 percent of the time worrying that only Nancy would show up, and if that turned out to be the case, quitting running altogether was the leading option. I wasn't going one on one with the powerbabe.

The run also fit in nicely with the Document's stated fifty-minute training time for week thirteen, session one. I figured it would take around forty-five minutes to complete the 5K run.

So all in all, it promised to be a good psychological and physical test that I looked forward to. Well, maybe I looked forward to it a bit too much since the night before produced one of my worst nights of sleep ever. Tossing and turning, then getting up and changing, over and over again. I was going to wear my running shorts for the first time, and I was struggling big time with going Pete McMartin kiltish style or staid, conservative Stanfield style. Oh, the pressure and pain McMartin and that sales representative had exerted upon me by suggesting there was an underwear option was torturous. By the end of the night I think it was the Stanfield style that won out, but only because that's what I woke up in.

I put on the rest of my running gear, drank some coffee, then woke up Shelly and Emma when I accidentally kicked over the painted pile of wood while stretching my calf muscles. After I made my way out the door, a massive attack of self-doubt kicked in as my knees started knocking against each other. My walk to McKitrick Park became a death march while I tried to convince myself that my knees were shaking not because I was scared silly but because it was a bit frosty out.

Once I got a sightline on the park, I was never so happy to see a crowd of people in my whole life. I wasn't sure what excuse I would have used if only Nancy and I had shown up, but stepping in front of, well, anything that moved was not out of the question. In actual fact, the opposite situation occurred; there were lots of people milling about, but no sign of Nancy.

While standing inside the ice rink in the registration line, I kept one eye out for Nancy and two ears open for the stories going on around me. It seemed I wasn't the only one suffering from a touch of anxiety. Different groups of people were milling about, asking where the route was, where the registration line was, and where the washrooms were. As it turned out, this was the first ever Run for Life event, which more than anything was the source of all of the confusion. People simply hadn't been to this run before. I found myself feeling more at ease when I started answering some of the questions. I knew where the washrooms were, and I knew which line was for registering names in the first half of the alphabet and which one was for the second half of the alphabet since I had arrived when the lineups were smaller and the signs were still visible.

My self-satisfaction came to a halt once I was registered and handed a plastic bag containing pamphlets and promotional nutritional bars that weighed in at about a pound. I twisted and turned through the throng of entrants until I was back outside, where I stood dumbfounded. What in the world was I going to do with all this marketing material? I cursed my inability to imagine the possibility of this predicament. I held the pamphlets up, rolled them, folded them, then looked longingly to the parking lot just in case I had brought my car but had somehow forgotten about driving it there.

It then dawned on me that I should put the material in the pocket at the back of my jacket, which was normally reserved for folding the jacket in on itself. After a few frenetic Rubik's cube moves, the bag was jammed in the back of the jacket and I was back to feeling pleased about my situation. Of course, that lasted until I heard a loudspeaker announcing that we should all move to the north side of the ice rink to do our warm-up exercises. I remember thinking that this was all a little fast, wasn't it? I mean, couldn't we all just slow down a bit?

I dutifully walked around the corner, the marketing material spanking me all the way, then received the biggest shock of the morning. There was Nancy, fully energized as she synchronized her body movements to a loud rock and roll track. Oh, there were some other aerobic leaders up on the steps for us to follow, but I had eyes only for Nancy. What was going on here—mother, part-time worker, Sun Run participant, Sun Run Team Leader, Run for Life participant, and now aerobic leader? This woman was an indomitable force; it appeared that she did it all.

My attempt to follow Nancy's lead lasted, oh, thirty seconds as it became painfully obvious I was going to bruise myself with the big whack of paper I had swinging around in the back of my jacket. I feigned a few groin stretches while the masses jumped for joy, then started to sweat when I realized that running with the back pocket full was a no go. The darn bag had me lost in thought, so I didn't hear the call to charge towards the big electronic timing clock set up at the crosswalk to Berm's Peak. I had been left behind, yet I made no attempt to make up the lost ground. Instead, I moved out towards the ice rink.

Oh, I wasn't quitting—that would have been far too easy—but I did have to deal with the cargo issue. Once inside the ice rink corridor, where I had decided to return the plastic bag to its original location at the registration table, a young voice from behind a counter to my left said, "Check your bag, sir?" Using a bag check was much more civilized than my initial plan, so I unloaded my burden then took advantage of the absence of a lineup and made my way to the washroom. I attained triple relief when I exited the ice rink doors and saw the backs of two hundred people moving out down 111th Street. Thank goodness, because I hadn't really wanted to work up the jam to mix and jostle at the start line with so many shiny happy people, with their endorphins redlining and all, if it wasn't necessary.

Regardless of my sentiments, it didn't take long before I caught up to a group of walkers on 111th Street. Now this is going to be hard to believe, but I pulled back on the throttle a bit here. The conversation between two women in their late twenties was too good to pass up. The two were accusing a third, who was not present, of having stolen every last stitch of clothing that she had worn while out bar-hopping with them the previous night. When I heard one of them say, "At least it was coordinated," I smiled and picked up the pace.

222

My interest was piqued by the next set of walkers as well, but when I wanted to get chatty and add my opinion to the conversation, I realized how unfocused I was on the task at hand and once again pushed on. I was struck by how many walkers I was passing and how good of a time they all seemed to be having. My naïveté knew no bounds.

There was a Run for Life volunteer course marshal directing us to turn right on 82nd Avenue, just as an organizer said there would be. Thank goodness, because until I saw the gentle windmill of his arms, my successful completion of the event had been in doubt. This is because I'm one of those people who get lost quite easily. I can say "those people" with the complete confidence of knowing others exist because I married one. Shelly and I both have high expectations that when Emma grows up she will excel in orienteering and be our guiding light, at least out to the new Ikea.

A strange thing happened, apart from nearly hypnotizing myself on the volunteer's whirling arm. I got passed. The strange part was that walkers passed me. Oh, they were running at the time, but when I had passed them they had been walking. As I was figuring this out, a party of three women (one pushing a baby buggy) stopped running in front of me and I passed them. It was as if I was caught up in the machinations of an intricate shuttle system, where various parts were doing random-length run/walk sessions.

While I was figuring out whether it was only a matter of time before each and every walker used me as passing fodder, it caught my attention that maybe the machine was breaking down. It seemed that everybody was walking on the slight grade of 82nd Avenue towards the North Delta High School. The runners immediately ahead of me were cutting out and walking. Whoa. That was unexpected, but before I could take any satisfaction in this observation, the party of three women (with one pushing a baby buggy) were running again—and of course passing.

The buggy party of three passed, huffing and puffing, then settled in front of me as they hunkered down to make it up the increasingly steep grade. Within seconds if not milli-seconds, the buggy party slowed its pace, and we all became part of a tightly packed group.

The woman pushing the buggy had red hair and a lithe runner's body that was taller than mine. She was on my left, while directly in front of the buggy was a smaller woman, Shelly size, with shoulder-length dark blonde hair in a ponytail that she had fitted through the back of her cap. The third woman, who was inches in front of me, had Scandinavian blonde hair and looked to be the same height or an inch taller than I was. They all wore form-fitted Lycra running gear with the unfettered style and grace of, well, someone with no body issues, and of course they were all twenty-nine.

Although the bevy of beauties was pleasant enough from a visual perspective, the situation was as far removed from the Sungod Track as one could get. I was physically restricted, I was fearful of tripping, and in my state of respiratory overexertion I was dreadfully aware of each and every Hoover-sucking, mouth-gaping inhalation and every nostril-flaring, horse-snorting exhalation that emanated from each of us. I would have snapped on a signal light and pulled out if I could have, but the grade of the street made any thought of that preposterous. Instead, all four of us were in staying-alive mode as we grunted on.

Salvation lay outside the North Delta High School in the form of a water station. I knew from my extensive grade research that this was the highest point in the neighbourhood. I had my sights set a touch over the Scandinavian blonde's shoulder on a paper cup of water, sitting on a table sixty feet away, when it was unceremoniously grabbed from view. I adjusted my sightlines to over the other shoulder and followed the arc of the cup as it tilted and drained, much to my chagrin, right into Nancy's gullet.

This was the last thing I wanted to happen: me passing Nancy. I was about to pass out from the stress of this complex happenstance, but before I could fabricate an alternate medical emergency exit, I watched

Nancy chuck the cup down and take off with renewed purpose. The buggy party of three stopped at the water table, while I grabbed a cup on the run.

I carried the water a bit farther without drinking because I was petrified that Nancy would suddenly stop and I would slingshot past her while I casually drank my water. It would be the equivalent of Pete McMartin passing me with his scarf in full bloom. It wasn't until she had passed a few runners and widened the gap between us that I dared take a sip. I had no idea where the route would take us, but I knew this was either the flat or even the downhill portion of the run, so I finished the water and relaxed a bit. Minutes later we were running southbound on 116th Street, and once we crossed 80th Avenue it was all downhill, which posed my next biggest problem. Oh, it had nothing to do with Nancy—thankfully, she was still widening the gap between us—but it had everything to do with another runner.

I could not believe my eyes. I was closing down hard on the back of a heavy-set, balding, middle-aged man who wasn't walking, limping, or in mid–heart attack. In fact, once I got past the unsightly dark stain down the back of his grey sweatshirt, I could see that he had a pretty fine running form but happened to be decelerating while I was accelerating. I weaved to one edge of the concrete runway, then to the other edge as I tried to figure out which side of the sidewalk to pass him on. My speed (yes, my speed) made the final determination; the gap became too narrow to weave again, so I passed him on the second weave, which was on his left side.

I could feel my centre of gravity rise to my hat for the brief moment that we were shoulder to shoulder, making me vulnerable to any skulduggery that I associated with my previous athletic endeavours. You know, like a lightning-quick Gordie Howe elbow that would end the pass and quite possibly my running career in mid-stride. So to counteract the light-headedness and the potential act of male aggression, I picked up the pace and can say that my first ever pass of a runner was an old-fashioned blowout.

I made a quick search downstreet for Nancy, and when I
determined that the gap was still getting larger, I had to force myself
not to turn and look over my shoulder to see whom exactly I had
passed. I never did do the Landy left shoulder check, not because of
any sense of decorum or fair play, but because I was back to emergency
stations again and had to keep my eyes and a full level of concentration
ahead of me, not behind. You see, the buggy party of three were
running again, and they did the usual by passing and pulling into a
tight formation. I must have been a moving goalpost for them to set
their sights on and surge ahead of, then catch their breath during the
now inevitable retreat. Sort of the opposite of my plan of action for
Nancy.

We all took up the same positions, with me being boxed in good
and tight by the buggy on my left and various track barriers of cedar
hedges, fir trees, and fences on my right. The gentle downward slope
that we were running made the adjustment to the tight quarters much
easier this time.

Without the strain of staying alive on a steep grade, I was able
to appreciate some of the finer points of the running group. My eyes
wandered to a particular piece of yellow polymer fabric that fit so
snugly I had to look twice just to make sure it wasn't paint. The soft,
graceful bend that the waterproof material took belied the strong, firm
frame beneath it. The shocks attached to the tubular titanium frame
allowed the buggy to move as if in a slipstream whenever its wheels
touched the grassed edges of the sidewalk. The wheels were something
else, chrome spokes attached to chrome rims that effortlessly turned
fat air-inflated tires. I was amazed. I hadn't known such marvel of
automotive engineering had trickled down to the baby buggy.

I was temporarily distracted by the rapid swinging of the dark
blonde's ponytail, and when I looked up I could see that she was turning
her head every once in a while to glance at the Scandinavian blonde,
then to look back at me. She had what I thought to be a mischievous, I-
know-something-you-don't-know look in her eyes, but I had to take one

more look at the buggy before I gave the meaning of her darting eyes my full scrutiny. You see, there was a problem with the buggy. Like, where was the baby? I could see water bottles, at least one maple-leaf-red track suit, a sweater, hats and wallets, woolen gloves, headphones, and the white plastic bags containing the marketing material, but where on earth was the baby? My conclusion was that there wasn't a baby. This group of friends treated their running experience in much the same fashion as one would a camping trip, and the buggy wasn't much more than a wheelbarrow.

My thoughts had drifted to *This is the type of preparedness that Canadian Girls In Training would have* when things went awry and I had to rely on my own training preparedness. It started with a deep, raspy double cough followed by the silky sensation of the Scandinavian blonde's hair covering my face as she threw her head back. My heart must have skipped a beat at the darkness of it all, but then I saw the light when her head shot forward under the propulsion of yet another wicked hack. In a forceful manner, her rear end jutted backwards, causing me to spoon her slender physique for fear of being accused of rutting her to the ground.

As it turned out she was going down anyway, which brought about my next dilemma: pits or breasts. If I chose pits, there was the possibility that the higher pick-up point might not break her fall. I knew if I dove in and grabbed her by her breasts it would be a sure catch based on the lower, wider body point, which would also give me a larger margin of error. In the end, the prudish law-abiding side of my character came out and I just couldn't do the public breast grabbing, so I did a Toller Cranston hand roll and took her off my shoelaces by the pits.

It was a stunning display of athleticism, after which I brought her narrow shoulders to an upright position, from where she turned her head sideways and placed her warm cheek against mine. Now, I wasn't expecting a tender look into my eyes accompanied by a "Thanks, I needed that," but I wasn't expecting her cheek to swell against mine and then to feel the pressure release of what turned out to be a hurling green phlegm ball, either. We continued to run cheek to cheek while we watched her sputum pass through an "as seen on TV" circular Stargate explosion. It wasn't until the ball cleared a wooden red-stained fence that I took my hands from her pits and in successful clutch-catch tradition licked the tips of my fingers.

I still had my tongue out when a high-pitched scream made me look in the pony-tailed woman's direction. Everything was open about her: her jacket, her hands, her eyes, her mouth, and her embarrassment as she looked first at me and then at her ominously silent friend. Before I could withdraw my exposed taste buds, hysterical laughter broke out among the three of them, and they bolted from view when they turned right on 75A Avenue. A few steps later I was turning right, and I too had a loud belly laugh going. A volunteer course marshal around the corner was scratching his head because he had the misfortune of witnessing the laughter but not seeing any of the action.

Although the buggy party of three had left me in the dust, the laughter left me refreshed and ready to take on the final quarter of the run now that its participants had strung out along the course with a quick succession of rights and lefts.

I rounded the corner at the south end of Swanson Drive and saw two other runners on the steepest grade I had ever set my running sights upon. At mid-grade was a young woman who appeared to be struggling, and at the top of the grade was Nancy. I did the math on a few worst-case scenarios, and euphoria set in once I figured it was impossible to catch Nancy. I then hooked a look at the mid-grade runner and began to reel myself up the street. The competitive spirits oozed out of all my pores as I closed within three feet of the woman, who seemed to be swaying gently in her stride as we hit the top of the grade. But three feet was as close as I got because once the route turned left at 78th Avenue and flattened out, she unleashed a storage of energy that propelled her out of range.

With McKitrick Park in sight at the end of the street, I thought of matching the runner's energy reserve, but it really wasn't an option. I had entered the Run for Life race with the goal of being consistent by finishing as strongly as I had started, and that was how I entered into McKitrick Park via the entranceway boulevard. Well, that's my story for running out of gas, and I'm sticking to it.

Shelly and Emma met me on the wrong side of the clock, and I had to first coax then shepherd them along in some strange circle dance for the last fifty feet. As I was crossing the finish line with my reluctant entourage, I heard my name being called out over the public address system. I can only hope they were saying nice things, but because of the cacophony created by previous runners at the finish area and the slight muffling of the announcement, they could have just as easily been scolding me for my apparent revelry on the track. Once again, crowd control was an issue on the Sungod Track.

When I crossed the finish line I had pushed the stop button on my wristwatch, which had a greater degree of accuracy than the Run for Life timer since I hadn't started the race when the official timer was set. The thirty-five-minute result for five kilometres left me a bit stunned once I pro-rated it and compared it with my first ten-kilometre timing of eighty-eight minutes. I remember wanting to talk about my oh so glorious speed but found myself standing alone, leaving me to enhance the legend in my mind without spousal contestation. Shelly and Emma had sauntered away with Nancy and her daughter to line up for the children's one-kilometre run, one lap around the Sungod Track.

I turned my face to the sun, closed my eyes, and began the wait for my family's return. I was reviewing the entire race, and I felt a tinge of pain in my lower back when I got to the part where running became a contact sport. The palms of my hands found their way to the small of my back, and I did a small series of stretches. *Oh, no,* I thought. My back had been fair to good in recent years, but it was a shoestring catch that had started my back problems many years ago.

At that moment my concerns began to mount over whether another shoestring catch had re-initiated the pain process. The sympathy-pain angle was being trial fitted on a short list of possibilities when I was interrupted by a familiar male voice.

I opened my eyes to see a young engineer from the factory where I used to work and his attractive wife. After a quick "How are you?" and once I determined that he was an experienced runner after we traded race finish times, the conversation itself became a race, but this time for information. First up I wanted to know what he thought about the hills and the length of the course. When he mentioned that he usually ran for eight kilometres with a running group that met at McKitrick Park, I wanted to know all about the group. Then I told him I trained here on the L shaped track and that it was elevated on each end, making 50 percent of the track uphill. The engineer stopped talking and did his best Clint Eastwood squint as he surveyed the landscape.

When he completed the survey, he said he had heard two other runners from his group talking about the park, saying it was named after a William McKitrick who had farmed the land in the years following World War II. Years after learning this, I had the good fortune to talk to Frank McKitrick of Penticton, a nephew of the North Delta farmer.

Frank told me he had often visited his Uncle Bill on the chicken farm while growing up and that he later worked on the farm, repairing wooden boxes that were obtained from the local farm markets. The boxes were then sold back to local farmers, who used them to bring their product to the market. Uncle Bill was a World War II veteran who had been wounded in the back during the battle of Dunkirk. My own Irish/Scottish heritage is similar to Uncle Bill's, as he was born in the Glasgow suburb of Lark Hall to parents of Irish descent. Frank said his Uncle was a proud veteran who participated in the Legion up to his death in 1990 and that he is buried in the White Rock Veterans Cemetery.

Moments later, Emma came running hard down the track and ran smack into my leg, signalling the end of her race. "Where's your momma?" I asked. She hugged me tightly and gave no reply since she was out of breath. I had to scan way back on the track to see Shelly running out of the woods, taking a shortcut through the parking lot. Her long hair swung one way while her unzipped rainwear swung another way, and under each arm she held a bundle of woolen clothing; when one bundle flapped, the other twirled vibrant colours. She moved in all known dimensions of space at once. I would tell her about the baby buggy trick later.

Within minutes the engineer, his wife, my wife and daughter, and Nancy and her daughter were all standing together on the grassed roundabout outside the ice rink. I suppose I knew that everyone wanted to leave, but my conversation was nowhere near an end as I delved into the experienced runner's Sun Run history. Nancy took charge of the situation and butted in to ask if I had picked up my prize. When I told her I had no idea if I had won or not, she took the number off my shirt, walked over to the rink, then came back with my prize: a gift certificate for a haircut from the salon I happen to go to. The prize hand-off ended the conversation, and we began the walk home.

The Sun Run training Document honed its continuous improvement aspect based on feedback from thousands of runners. Nancy and I added our two cents to the accrued knowledge as we talked about our success and a job well done on the way home. Although Nancy had been training with the Sungod Sun Run training clinic and could test herself against other runners, I got the feeling that she had needed this race as much as I had. The Document had prepared the both of us physically, but it was now up to us to make it a lock in our minds that we were capable—I mean really capable—of, well, as the Document said, "See you at the finish line."

Session 2   40 minutes. Run 40 minutes. Tuesday, April 1, 2003.

I had been looking forward to this training session for thirteen weeks. This was the Document's last scheduled training session, and because of that I was determined to make a good showing of it. The run took place in the mid-afternoon on a perfect Pacific Northwest spring day. I had the doors and windows open while I did my warm-up exercises and made the decision (without any of the usual first-time anguish) to not wear my running jacket. Wearing running shorts for the first time during the Run for Life had worked out so well that I felt comfortable making another big change with the jacket.

Oh, I considered these to be big changes, not only from a physical point of view but from a superstitious one as well. I know I've mentioned that I wore golden cleats in the past, but not why. The reason is very simple. I wore them because they were a part of my lucky attire. Yes, I believe that luck comes into play in many different ways. In the old days (you know, pre-calculator let alone personal computer), I had a lucky black dickie. When the dickie was on it was win at all costs, but of course back in those days blowing out a knee or having a heart attack weren't considered viable expenditures. The dickie and any vespers of its significance are long gone from my competitive spirit, thank goodness, and I keep luck on my side in different ways now, such as in paying homage to Poh-Poh.

Left behind were the jacket and long sweatpants as I hit the street running on a meticulously timed and measured route worthy of a Municipality of Delta surveyor certificate. My objective in creating an off-track running route was to incorporate some of the conditions that made the Sungod Track so successful. So in keeping with Berm's Peak at the north end of the Sungod Track and Lesser Berm's Peak behind the Sungod Pool, I picked two grades that were in proportion to the five-kilometre circular track. The lesser grade was from the willow tree, then over to and up 80th Avenue to 116th Street. The steeper of the two grades was from 72nd Avenue northward along 112th Street, which ended at the entrance to the Sungod Recreation Centre. The route was mostly cement, with half a kilometre on asphalt, and like the Sungod Track was 50 percent uphill.

All was well until I got to the final leg of the route on 112th Street, which was three decimal points over one kilometre in length, all uphill. I had pretty much lost count of how many times I had tripped the odometer button on this grade. So I had seen it many times from the driver's seat, but it's not until you round the corner from 72nd Avenue and see it from a runner's perspective that the feeling of having bitten off more than you can chew enters into your mind. It was also at this point that the new reference track got its name, the Sungod Crest. I had originally called the route Oliver's Run after the Delta resident and former premier of British Columbia. His surname adorned 112th Street before the municipality of Delta switched over to the numeric street-naming system. But when my eyes focused on the crest of land that ended the grade at the Sungod Recreation Centre reader board, the route's rightful name became evident.

I began the challenge with the customary Toller Cranston hand roll and a fine-tuning of my posture (you know, chin up and the whole bit). This grade represented the Document's conclusion to my Sun Run training program of thirteen weeks, thirty-eight training sessions, two hundred and seventy-three run/walk segments. There was no way I was going to pull up short, pare my effort, or truncate this session in any manner and cast a pall of doubt over the effectiveness of the program.

Having said that, I almost stopped dead in my tracks less than one minute into the ascent. The view was breathtaking. It was of a view corridor I'd never seen before because I normally approach the busy intersection of 72nd Avenue and 112th Street in my car, and my concentration would be on the task at hand—negotiating the traffic— and so I would pass the view unseen. Then again, it's not as if I hadn't seen Burns Bog from 72nd Avenue, but this was a different perspective that included portions of the San Juan and Gulf Island chains. On my port side one block north was 72nd A Avenue, which showcased Orcas Island to the left and Salt Spring Island behind Point Roberts on the right, with the bog of course providing a lush green foreground.

Although there were still hours of sunlight left, the sun was on a shallow early-spring trajectory, which would have it set directly behind the vista, making it worthy of taking a seat on one of the neighbour's lawns and taking it all in—if I had been on vacation. Of course, I wasn't on vacation, so I swung my head around and looked for the Sungod Crest but failed to capture it because of yet another gorgeous view. You would have thought it was my first time to this part of Delta, but with the cold, clear atmosphere and the spotlight effect of the early spring sun, the focus of Seymour Mountain was so crisp it looked as if it were an extension of the Sungod Crest. Although it was this deception that enhanced the mountain's aesthetic beauty, it still was a striking sight that filled me with wonder. A few steps later common sense prevailed and said that the mountain's eastern slope continued past the Sungod Crest and slipped into the calm shoreline of Indian Arm.

Because of the grade, it didn't take long before my eyebrows were topped with sweat, which in turn fogged my eyeglasses. With the beauty of my distant visions a blur, I was reduced to staring down the stark, solemn outlines of the telephone poles. I began to worry because it was early into the grade and I could feel myself slowing with each step. I didn't need to do much calculating to figure out that at the rate I was going, I would come to a complete stop, oh, probably within spitting distance.

I did an extended Toller Cranston hand roll, leaving my fingers outstretched while I stared down the nearest telephone pole until it had completely left my field of vision. When the pole was behind me I completed the hand roll, then stretched the fingers out again while I fixated on the next pole. The sensation of passing the poles in this manner was like blowing by them at highway speeds. Oh, it felt good. I continued with this pole-to-pole racing until I was faced with an unprecedented challenge just short of the crest outside Burnsview school.

The sounds were hideous, the sight was abhorrent and my response was instantaneous and menacing in nature. I guess school was out, and a group of about six skater boys came upon me as they exited the front doors. They all groaned, moaned, and made death wails worthy of any junior high stage play as they did a quick jog to catch up to me on the sidewalk. Topped with their domed baseball caps on sideways and anchored by stiff, baggy-legged pants, they looked like a group of bowling pins as they swayed and crooned in unison before me. They could have been from the track class I had seen in the past, but I didn't recognize them in their after-school get-ups, just as I'm sure they didn't recognize me in mine (sans the little white dog).

Whatever the case, I was having none of their impetuous and insolent action; I stuck my arm out, locked at the elbow, and gave them the unsanctioned Elvis Stojko kung-fu-style fingers to open palm wave. It was like *Bring it on*, then I turned it on (you know, picked the speed up maybe point zero, zero, zero one faster per kilometre up the steepest part of the grade). The skater boys scrambled to catch up and pass me before they splayed themselves about a bus-stop bench and brought the vocalization process to a crescendo as I passed them. Oh, there were a few pins left standing when I passed, but I could see them wobble, even if it was in laughter, as they left my field of vision.

I admired the stopped time of forty minutes on my wristwatch during the cool-down walk from the willow tree back to the house since it was exactly what the Document had ordered. My revelling in the good fortune of the final five-kilometre timing came to a sudden and unexpected end when I saw Shelly's nail-polish-red SUV in the driveway. My pace quickened and my heart raced in anticipation of seeing my wife, but when I rounded the corner to the back door I took in a rather large whiff of cigarette smoke and let out an involuntary gasp that somehow had a farm animal resonance to it.

"You leave Pete McMartin and me out of this. If we want to smoke and run we damn well will, you hear me?" said Shelly as she sat in her powder-blue running wear on the stairs leading to the back door.

Nothing like getting off on the wrong foot. I wanted so much to say that I had no idea if McMartin smoked. Besides it wasn't as if I was accusing him of pulling an Edmund Whitty. Whitty is a newspaper journalist who starts his day off with a teaspoon of alcohol mixed with a dash of cocaine, a pinch of marijuana, and a measure of opium. The ingredient quantities of the concoction are my own dipsomaniacal estimations.

I would have liked to have brought west coast author John MacLachlan Gray's fictional character into the conversation—you know, for much-needed whimsy—but I thought better of it. After all, it was only a few weeks ago that Denny Boyd was off limits, but it was all right to take a poke at McMartin. I remember thinking that there must be a whole heap of trouble going on if she was now defending McMartin, so I placed my hands over my head and tried to sneak sideways by her without making another sound. I got as far as the open back door when a force field was executed, from hinge plate to door jamb, when I heard "Your sister phoned." I chose the lesser of two evils and slowly backed up and sat in a plastic lawn chair at the foot of the stairs. It was a phone call I did not want to make.

Knowing what was about to come I crossed my legs at the ankle, folded my hands on my stomach, pursed my lips, and stared at the long-necked Mexican beer that Shelly was taking a swig from. I could see the sweat on the bottle but strangely none on Shelly, who I could tell had been out running because her cheeks were flushed. I wanted to ask why she was home early. I wanted to ask about her run, which had to have been incredibly short. I wanted to ask why she was now a McMartin defender, but in the end I held still and let the sun beat down on me while I watched the bottle intently. Oh, it wasn't that I wanted a drink, it was just that I wanted *that* drink, and when Shelly began talking again after another puff on her cigarette, I imagined holding the long-necked bottle as a cold compress and rolling it ever so gently up and down the inside of my aching right knee.

"I looked at your little piece of paper. You're finished, Dave. You don't have any excuses. Okay, you go to the doctor, then you don't have any excuses," said Shelly.

My fingers, ankles, and lips began to fuse as I attempted to ellipsis my way through the conversation, knowing that my will power would dissolve the instant I opened my mouth. I watched Shelly drink and smoke some more all the while hoping that she was well stocked. Then before the cigarette was anywhere near what I would call finished she snubbed it out and said, "you go tomorrow." Oh I didn't want to go anywhere so the two of us sat in the sun in silence. There was a clunk of an empty bottle hitting the wooden stairs and while I wished with all of my might that she would get up and get another she instead held her ground then pointed her finger at me and said, "you, you must face the music and dance."

I couldn't help myself the words just blurted out: "Arnold Schwarzenegger?" All I got was a giggle and a smile in return. "Tony Soprano? James Cagney? Bruno Gerussi?" I told her I was guessed out, which brought about more giggles and another rendition of some tough guy telling me I must dance. Being far too pleased with herself, Shelly got up off the stairs, adjusted her running wear, and told me it was based on the Irving Berlin song "Let's Face the Music and Dance."

My sister, the de facto family leader, phoned from Winnipeg minutes later. All my responses began and ended with the word *yes*. It seemed that all of Shelly's responses for the rest of the night began with *you* and ended with *dance*. There was very little sympathy for a guy with a fear of flying who was going to visit his hospitalized mother in Winnipeg.

Session 3   1st extra run before the Sun Run, 25 minutes. Thursday, April 3, 2003.

My doctor, who was also my dad's doctor, knows I'd spent all my adult life working in the aviation industry. He always asks me the same question when we get on the subject of my fear of flying, or as I refer to it, my preference not to fly. He is never on the other side of his desk when he asks it, he is never occupied with putting away some medical apparatus, he is never looking at my chart. Instead, he is always standing face to face when he unleashes the full baritone of his query: "Is there something I should know?" I always laugh but often wonder if he is imploring me to whisper some dark trade secret. It would be nice if the answer could be neatly tied up in some technical manner such as corrosion, but the problem lies with the paradigm of my common sense, not the aircraft.

Anyway, I didn't go to the doctor before this trip, not because I wasn't in a laughing mood but because I hadn't fully recovered from my last flight, which was out of Los Angeles a few weeks after the September 11, 2001, terrorist attacks. Since this isn't a story about assault rifles, air marshals, or onboard fisticuffs, I'll move on to my final run before I boarded a bus to Winnipeg.

Shock of shocks, the Document did not lead into the Sun Run after its last training session. I had trouble with this, first because I was disappointed in myself for not seeing the time gap, and second, I now had to think up two schedules. Yes, one schedule for me and the other for Shelly, whose last words before she exited the door for her training runs were always spoken in true game-show-host fashion, "Give me some numbers." Since she had stopped carrying the stopwatch long before and had never worn a watch while running, who knows what good my numbers would be, but I gave honest numbers anyway.

As far as numbers for me, I had no idea. The Document had abandoned me at the bottom of a training ramp-down at forty minutes.

I didn't know whether to ramp up, and if so to what, or to maintain the shorter run times before the main event of the Sun Run. For Shelly's numbers, I had some personal history to work with, but for my numbers I was clueless, so I went with the easy route of what the body craved—which wasn't necessarily what the body needed. The Sungod Crest run had sapped my body of energy, so I planned an easy run of about forty minutes on an all-flat surface that was soft to boot. I figured the forty minutes represented a trickle charge, so to speak, the flatness a treat, and the fact that I would run on a different route with a soft surface was downright clever on my behalf (you know, good for the body and soul).

I thought I would run the Burns Bog trail again, but this time from 72nd Avenue towards the Alex Fraser Bridge. So the post-Document era was going to start off with something new and refreshing, including the timing of it all. I planned to take a page out of Shelly's running repertoire and run free by leaving the watch at home.

My version of casual run day started off all downhill in a light drizzle on 112th Street as I made my way to hooking up with the Bog Trail under the 72nd Street overpass. I had never been here before. I had always started the trail from the Alex Fraser Bridge end and never walked or even ran as far as 72nd Avenue, although last time I had come close enough to hear the traffic before turning back.

On my way to the trail I compiled a list of things to do before I left later that evening. After packing my runners, the list was pretty much all literary related, from buying a cassette player to packing pens and paper. Previous bus or train excursions to Winnipeg, which included a couple of overnighters, taught me that reading a book was difficult because of the limited amount of light, so I was going the audiobook route this trip. Since I had finished the non-fiction Emily Carr memoir by Klee Wyck the night before, I decided that all the cassettes would be fiction. I would either borrow them from the library or in the case of one of my favourite authors, Douglas Coupland, I would make a purchase.

Once I got on the trail I was immediately taken back by the size of the trees. I was accustomed to the light, smooth skins of the spindly and tightly packed alders, but the trees at this end of the trail were enormous firs, sporting fibrous bark with furrows deep enough that I could put my entire fist in. The drizzle and traffic noise came to an abrupt stop, while the drop in temperature made me wish for my running jacket. The view of the trail was of a tunnel through a dark green forest that was flat and straight and had the finality of blackness as its destination. It wasn't until I took note of the dripping sounds all around me that I realized I was alone. I did a few shoulder checks, then even ran backwards for a bit to confirm my solitude, which did nothing to stop the developing shiver.

I began to question my lack of route vigilance and how I had let this happen, considering that comfort, security, and familiarity as found on the Sungod Track were the virtues I embraced. This casual run day and the ensuing twisting and turning had bunched my shorts, and that was before I looked down at my wrist to see the time. Not seeing my watch and not knowing my distance run based on an eight-minute kilometre added additional stress that somehow translated into faster-moving feet. Then a combination of moving through the urban wilderness at a pretty good clip and thinking about how Emily Carr survived long solo sojourns into British Columbia's lush rain forests to do her painting relaxed me to the point where running backwards wasn't necessary.

I was practicing deep breathing and perfect form as additional methods of banishing my fears when the run unravelled big time. Oh, I didn't need inner peace—what I needed at the time was a hand to hold onto or at the very least someone else on the trail, friend or foe. Instead all I had was me, myself, and a mind that derailed when it saw the railroad tracks.

It all began innocuously enough when I was working on my form. I saw the tracks at the bottom of the embankment on my left, then lost sight of them when a thicket of trees removed the image from view.

When the image reappeared a minute later, it brought with it a source of dread that put me into immediate orthographic viewing overload. In all my years of blueprint reading I had never subjected my skills to such intensive use. I took the image of the railway tracks and my position to them and twisted it and turned it and looked at it from one side then the other to no avail. I was lost. The tracks were my reference point, and they were indicating contrary information.

When I ran the bog trail last time, the tracks were on my left, so I figured at the beginning of this run from the opposite end the tracks should have been on my right, but no they were on my left. The chance of Burlington Northern moving them out of position overnight wasn't a possibility, so that meant I was out of position. By the time I had taken into account the bigger than usual trees, the projection screen had gone stark white.

It was then that I pushed myself over the top by imagining that the rustle behind me was D'Sonoqua, a supernatural being that lives in the forest. I had been reading about the Indian legend in the Emily Carr book the night before. She had said of one carved totem pole representation that horror tumbled out of the unfathomable shadows of its eye, cheek, and mouth. I had most likely produced enough adrenalin prior to introducing the Carr image to take action, but D'Sonoqua ensured that the toggle switch was set to the flee response rather than the fight or freeze.

I took the next path out of my predicament by turning right and running up the side of a steep embankment in a manic search for concrete and its accompanying civilization. On the third switchback I slowed a bit, not because my fear had subsided but because the path was a bit greasy from rain that had seeped through the overhead canopy of trees. On the sixth switchback I began to regret waking up that morning. On the seventh switchback I wanted to stop, but since I had never stopped once during any portion of my Sun Run training, I was having trouble coming to terms with doing it a first time. While I negotiated my release from my narcissistic obligations,

I pushed myself like a rented mule, only slower through the final two switchbacks.

I exited the woods and drew a bearing on a street sign on the far side of the street. I was steps away from reading the sign and attaining emotional relief when I heard "Nice day for a walk, eh?" I looked to the side and saw some old geezer stepping into his parked mid-seventies relic made from Detroit iron. I didn't respond, I couldn't. I was running for my life.

The sign said, "Monroe Drive and Barrymore Drive." I recognized Monroe as being the street running along the south end of the Sungod Track and felt that I had successfully rescued myself. As I looked up Monroe Drive I could see that the hellacious climb was far from over, but by then it wasn't as if I had a choice in quitting or not. So once I was out of the old geezer's sightline, I picked out a piece of grass to the side of the road and collapsed to my knees, which was then followed by a slow-motion face plant.

Oh, I'll remember that feeling for the rest of my life. The spring showers had turned the grass sod to a soft and watery mush, which turned out to be the requisite treatment for my desiccated internal organs. Within seconds I had sunk at least an inch into the ground, providing a head-to-foot sensation that produced a sob. Okay, two or three sobs. After that I was able to open one eye and check for witnesses through thick, sticky lashes and rain-laden strands of grass. Even with these impediments I somehow assured myself that I was alone, so I closed the eye and drifted unencumbered of human interaction to my thoughts of Cuyler Goodwill.

When Cuyler lay before his scale model of the Great Pyramid, he too surrendered himself to the earth as he focused his mind on his long-lost love. Carol Shields's depiction of this character's final moments on earth is one of the highlights of *The Stone Diaries*. My thoughts while I sank further into the sod were of the rewarding experience I had during my first reading of the novel as the resonate detail of Cuyler Goodwill's death emerged line by line, page by page, raindrop by raindrop. In particular I loved the fact that Cuyler had trouble remembering his lost love's name—I found it remarkably telling. I then remember thinking that I was feeling the same physical sensations Cuyler did when it dawned on me that Cuyler had died. It was with this sobering thought that I disengaged myself from Carol Shields's work and gathered myself for a lift. While I cleaned some mud out from behind my glasses and checked for wrinkling of the skin, I also kept my one good eye looking out for the Delta Police. I didn't want to explain myself, not any part of it.

The walk home was steep, very wet, and exhausting, but when I finally got there I didn't complete my run routine by showering and changing. Instead, I grabbed the car keys and rifled through the glove compartment to get my map. I needed to figure out how I had gotten lost. After studying the map something did not seem right, so I started up the convertible and drove down to the corner of Bates and Browning Drive, where I found problem number one: this corner does not exist. In all my years of getting lost this was a first; usually there is a street but no name on the map. Barrymore Drive was the last street to the trail that I had recently run on. It seemed that the trail, which was about a single lane wide, was called Browning Drive on the map, although there were no street signs confirming this.

I got out of the car with the map in hand, walked down to the trail, and kicked the dirt a bit. Sure enough, there was a rough layer of asphalt at my feet. The concealed Browning Drive turned trail made me wonder if I was in the Delta Bermuda Triangle, then I heard voices coming from the direction of the railway tracks. I scanned the area rapaciously in my quest for additional information, which came in the form of a man and woman walking a large unleashed dog on the far side of the tracks. The walkers showed me where in the landscape to focus on, and once I did this I recognized the Burns Bog trail immediately.

I stood for a while longer, looking out over the ravine with the railway tracks at the bottom, just sorting it all out. On one side of the tracks was a trail in the North Delta Nature Reserve, and on the other side was the Burns Bog trail; the two merge after the 72nd Avenue overpass to form a new trail leading to the Watershed Park at 64th Avenue. It couldn't be any more obvious as I stood there, but during the run it was all one wilderness.

The Winnipeg Trip

2nd extra run before the Sun Run. Saturday April 12, 2003

Shelly and Emma left me by myself on a hard bench in the stark confines of the New Westminster bus depot later that night after the North Delta Nature Reserve run. It took but a minute, but I chased after them once I had conducted a pungency analysis of the depot waiting room. I caught up to Shelly as she was backing out of her parking space, and the look on her face, as I signalled free form by the driver's side window, was as if she had just seen a madman.

"I need a smoke," I said once the window had powered down far enough to receive mail.

I'm not sure if she was being a good wife and a better friend or simply reacting in the involuntary manner of someone being robbed, but after reaching into her purse she pushed a fresh pack of cigarettes through the window opening, with no questions asked. A red lighter followed a moment later, then the window resealed itself with a certain exactness that made me purse my lips. I watched them drive through the poorly lit parking lot and saw the right back tire catch the curb as they cornered, then heard it squeal as it touched back down on the roadway. A sense of sadness settled in deeper than any Casablanca rerun; it didn't seem right to see them leave in such a hurry.

In this world there are bus passengers who are drivers and those who are non-drivers. Passengers who are drivers sit on the right side of the bus and drive vicariously every mile of their trip. I've seen passengers who are drivers get escorted off busses at 3:00 a.m. by the RCMP. They can be a freaky-deaky lot who drive themselves to exhaustion simply because they don't shift out like the professional drivers. I am a non-driving passenger, so when the bus came in I took a seat on the left side, window seat, mid-bus.

The trip was scheduled for forty-eight hours, so I took my time settling in, and it wasn't until we had left the Coast Mountain range behind that I pulled out my new cassette player and loaded an audiobook. Fumbling by moonlight, I found the play button and *Miss Wyoming* by Douglas Coupland opened with the narrator's soft feminine voice. I chose this audiobook without any investigation whatsoever into the dust-jacket blurb. I had walked down the aisle and grabbed it off the shelf without breaking stride based on the strength of the author's name.

I had become a huge fan of Douglas Coupland during the page turner of a novel *All Families Are Psychotic* when he introduced a secondary character by the name of "Shw." It was a moment of pop culture savvy that amused me to no end. Coupland then went on to fill out the female character with actions and dialogue that incredibly lived up to the name. This brought about a sense of realism that when mixed with my already piqued sense of humour made for a most satisfying reading experience.

In fact, having a character live up to a name is exactly what author Wayson Choy did with Poh-Poh. She was a diligent grandmother doting on the youngest of her grandchildren while forever espousing the ways of the old country to the older children. Her role of wise elder not only lived up to the name but also provided a cross-cultural reference. This enabled me, with my paternal third-generation northern Irish and maternal first-generation Scottish heritage, to identify in some small way with the Oriental character.

I bring up trying to identify with and understand the fictional character you know as opposed to the real characters on the bus because I was trying to find some common ground or some point of interest with the *Miss Wyoming* protagonist, Susan Colgate. Susan was a former beauty queen and failed actress. I've made it this far in life without the word *beauty* being associated with me, thank goodness— I have enough problems without having to carry beauty's matching baggage—but I have been told that I've been a bad actor on many occasions. These two elements of character creation came close, but nothing in the first five minutes of the story reached out and grabbed me.

Well, the second five minutes of the *Miss Wyoming* narration manhandled me then shook me to the core as the left engine blew on Susan's flight from New York to Los Angeles. As Coupland's story starts to describe the fate of the unbuckled passengers, I began a frantic search for my own seat belt in the dark cylindrical confines of my so-called preferred method of transportation. More than one sleepy head turned my way as I abandoned my search and thrashed about while opening a bottle of water, finally ending the fit by throwing the cassette player and headphones into the knapsack at my feet. I needed off that bus in the worst way. When a half-hour stop coincided with my catching the last drop of water on my tongue after one final death-do-us-part shake of the bottle, I considered it a sure sign that all would be well.

My staggered walk down the aisle went unnoticed, since everybody else seemed to be doing the same closing-hour dance from one row of seats to the next. Once outside, my hands did not fail me as they worked on the pack of cigarettes with the speed and dexterity of a bomb disposal specialist who has been told the final countdown had begun. When I got the soft wrap off and the hard cardboard box opened, I lifted my head and saw three young men, all about voting age. Without hesitation I gave each of them a cigarette, then I stuck out an unwavering hand for all to see and lit the cigarette of the one with the biggest potential to rant. Oh, I knew these three in as much as I knew (or at least made myself aware of) everyone on the bus. The one who had to stoop into the flame and another were friends who had boarded in a loud and obnoxious manner outside of Hope, B.C.

These rural boys were a couple of tall slim-jims who wore straight-legged jeans with plain, basic-coloured jackets. Both were hatless, exposing thick, unruly hairlines—logos and hairdressers need not apply. The third was heavyset and quiet, letting his clothing do all his talking. He was dressed as if he were a rap star who had the misfortune of stepping back onto the wrong tour bus. He sat in the same row as I did but on the other side of the aisle. I figured his bus screw-up originated at the New Westminster station.

After I lit the first slim-jim's cigarette, he took a drag and scrunched his face so tight that his lips looked like a wrinkled letter O. It was then that the first words were spoken by any of us. "You must be from Vancouver."

I gave the homosexual insinuation a simple "Yup" and began lighting the next filtered 100-millimetre, extra, extra light, menthol smoke with a five-syllable brand name that was pulled from the less popular twenty hard-pack. Soon we were all forming wrinkled O's and talking about Gulf War II. Well, I let the moochers talk about the war. I'd learned from previous Western Canadian bus excursions that the youth of today aren't interested in some paunchy older guy's predawn diatribe on international politics, only his cigarettes.

I once again bounced from one seat to the next on the way back to my non-driver's position, but for an entirely different reason. The cigarette had made me instantly sick to my stomach, which ended up being a good thing. You see, my writhing at least distracted me from converting my fear of flying into fear of bussing. With my arms holding my midsection, a voice murmured in the last moment before sleep that the second cigarette wouldn't be as painful Oh, addiction's vile whispers of assurance.

The bus pulled into downtown Winnipeg on schedule, and my only sibling, a younger sister named Meghan, picked me up. You can imagine after not shaving or bathing for two full days and then adding sleep deprivation and smelly decadent behaviour on top of it all, I must have looked worthy of being pushed back on the bus and sent on further East. Well, I did, but when I saw Meghan she looked worse. *Oh, for heaven's sake, Mum's dead,* I thought. Actually, I think this every single time I step off the bus or train in Winnipeg. Such is the nature of going incommunicado for two days. My mum's health problems, which began with polyarteritis nodosa when she was in her thirties, escalate thanks to my Poh-Poh–like predilection to look for signs of the worst-case scenario.

Meghan informed me that Mum's situation remained grave but that "she would still be available to tell me how nice it was of me to come, this time." It was easy to hold back a laugh since one did not form, but I sure have taken a lot of flack for not coming for a heart attack a few years back. Well, okay, I didn't come back for either one of them. Meghan has the best sense of humour in the family, the easiest laugh, and the keenest sense of humanity. Any of her friends will tell you that she is a wonderful conversationalist who has at one time or another helped them through tough times in their lives. But apart from the weak tossing of a line of parody followed by one short exhaustive breath, none of that was evident that day at the Winnipeg bus station.

On the drive to Meghan's home where I would wash up before visiting Mum at the hospital, I took note of the fact that she turned the radio off. Once at home I watched her casually walk by the radio in the kitchen, and with a flick of the wrist it too was off. By the time I finished up in the bathroom, the television, which had been left on by one of her grown children when we came in, was off as well.

I use music as an associative tool throughout my daily life, including common matters such as remembering the details about a person I haven't seen in a long time. I don't use it to remember names, but more for what that person was about—you know, what did they like as opposed to what were they like. So when music is used in a story it has an enormous impact on me. I know I would have fallen for Wayson Choy's character Poh-Poh without music, but when he brought a tidbit of it into *The Jade Peony,* he ensured that he not only had my heartstrings but also could play them like crazy, straight through to the story's end.

The clinching scene took place on a house porch in Vancouver's Chinatown, where Poh-Poh sat with her youngest grandson on her shoulder while she watched her eight-year-old granddaughter reach through the open picture window and place the turntable needle on an already spinning record. The song she chose was a traditional American folk song called "Shortnin Bread," which she did her best Shirley Temple tap dance routine to. I hummed that song through to the finish of the book. Then throughout my Sun Run training, because I was doing so much of the Poh-Poh cum Chicken Little the-sky-is-falling histrionics with regard to my physical health, "Shortnin Bread" was hummed often while I stepped gingerly around the Sungod Track.

Well, I took note of the music being turned off, but I failed to interpret the sign. Poh-Poh would have been disappointed in me. I should have recognized this sign of distress because the same thing happened to me after the World Trade Center buildings collapsed as a result of a terrorist attack; I didn't fire up the audio tubes for six straight weeks. So when I walked into the hospital room later that day, even after donning a paper face mask, I still was not tuned into the seriousness of the situation. Diverticulitis be damned, the moaning was unbearable. Meghan later explained—Mum sure wasn't doing any talking—that in the days leading up to entering the hospital, Mum's osteoporosis had weakened a vertebra to the point where it fractured, and that was the cause of the acute pain.

I could feel my own bones collapsing under my weight, and to break my fall I placed a hand on the nearest table. When the table began to roll I grabbed Meghan with the other hand and focused on the yellow do-not-resuscitate strap on Mum's wrist in order to regain my composure. The room spun, with a single static yellow dot at its centre . . . and then the coughing started. Great Scott, it was a room-shaking, pneumatic hack that halted the spin and had me convinced I was witnessing the final death rattle. I was dumbfounded when there was a respite in the cough and she was still alive, but when her next breath carried a low moan I made a soft exit. I never went back, but Meghan did—every day for ten months until Mum was released, albeit in a wheelchair because of muscular atrophy from being bedridden so long.

I spent the next several days talking to Meghan and trying to squeeze in a run. I wasn't successful for two reasons. First, I wasn't accustomed to the structure of the day. Meals were at odd hours, people came over unexpectedly, and there were phone calls at unusual times—in short, all the typical things that happen when you are out of town. The second reason was the most likely for not going for a run. I stepped out one morning under a clear deep blue sky, its captivating view of the sun unimpeded by mountains, smog, or architectural structures. I didn't need to take a second step to know it was just too darn cold.

My coldest day of training that winter had been zero Celsius, maybe minus one if you rounded down. On that morning it was minus three, and I could feel my skin tightening and my lungs burning before even getting down to business, so I put that run off until the afternoon. The problem with the afternoon was that it was too hot. The TV said it was plus nineteen Celsius, which was a no go for me. I had never trained even in the low teens let alone summer temperatures, and so because of the harsh conditions and my inability to schedule around them, I never trained while in Winnipeg.

Now I grew up in Winnipeg, so I knew all about minus thirty in the winter and plus thirty in the summer, but I had completely forgotten about the extreme temperature changes on any given day. The Greater

Vancouver winter/early spring temperature range was zero to plus twelve Celsius, while on any given day the change would be in the range of three to eight degrees. The temperature change of twenty-two degrees Celsius in Winnipeg while I was there in the spring of 2003 was downright beastly. I was disappointed in not running because I had been dreaming of running a prairie route with flatness all around. Flatness to the left, flatness to the right, flatness in each compass point. Oh, the glory of running on the flat.

It broke my heart to leave Meghan at the train station boarding area, but with no clear-cut indication of how and when the situation with Mum was going to resolve, I decided I had spent as much time as possible in Winnipeg. It also grieved me that in some small way I was leaving because I wanted to run the Sun Run, and this was the last train out of town that would get me back to Vancouver in time. Both Meghan and Shelly would have none of that nonsense of thought, but I still felt uneasy knowing the role it played as I settled into my economy coach seat.

I chose the train not because it was any faster than the bus, nor because I got a better sleep. I chose the train because of the food. You have to remember that I was in the final preparations for running in the Sun Run, so nutrition was on my mind and so was the fact that it would be eight days of not running after this trip. All through my training the longest I had gone between punching the run ticket was three days. I mostly trained every second day, and the thought of going eight days was a confidence destroyer. At that point I took solace in the fact that I hadn't registered. Really, what if I had lost it? What if I had to start over? Oh, the horror.

Twenty-four hours later, I was having a smoke in the 1950s art deco–style lounge railcar because I'd run out of French stories. You see, there was this young Australian woman sitting across the aisle from my seat in the adjoining car who was completely bonkers for everything French. I must admit there was a real French-Canadian flavour to our car, with the onboard attendant giving instructions in both French and English, and I could hear at least five different French conversations in the rows behind me. So the Aussie quizzed me with a straightforwardness and an eagerness on all things French by virtue of the fact that I was sitting closest to her. Fortunately for her, the powerbabe's daughter had been enrolled in French immersion since kindergarten, so I'd been brushing up on the basics over the years whenever she was at our house playing with Emma.

I gave the Aussie a few words—all with a Danny Gallivan inflection—a few Festival du Voyageur stories, then a few Louis Riel statue stories, but that was it. I was spent. I took refuge in the lounge rail car directly behind ours. I sat on the vinyl-tufted bench seat enjoying the solitude, which was enhanced by the black of night against the stainless steel framed windows. I figured I would review the Sun Run course, which I had read was the second year for this particular route.

The route had been clipped to the side of the fridge for months, right next to the Document, and sometimes right on top of or even clipped to the Document. Such is the electromagnetic meandering of a fridge door's life. I had not only memorized the route, but because I once lived central to it I had bussed, driven, and walked every portion of the route many times. With my arms extended on each side of the bench to attain maximum sprawl, I began at the start on Georgia Street until the scurrying feet of a man and a woman interrupted my contemplation. They darted one way through the car, then minutes later the other way before making their retreat, all the while cursing about their lost friend, whom I would meet soon enough.

To my utter amazement I noticed some movement at floor level, about the shape and consistency of a cat, then the hairball rose and a head emerged from under a table on the other side of the car. The head, with its gaping mouth in a full drop-down position, then let out a groggy four-letter expletive. It was Ricky, who had folded himself head-to-ankle scissors-like and passed out. It was the most peculiar thing to think that I had been alone, apart from the serene crowd up

253

in the domed observation level, only to have a piece of the furniture come to life. Moments later, before Ricky could even acknowledge he was on a train let alone that I was sitting in front of him, Julian and Bubbles came in and found him.

Okay, so I had given them names after the television show *Trailer Park Boys*. They were a drunken crew who were travelling from the Maritimes to Calgary, seven in all, including one set of parents, Julian's. By the time I had caught up to them in Winnipeg they had been cut off alcohol by the onboard staff, oh, somewhere in Ontario, which only gave them the green light to drink their own booze, morning, day, and night. Finding Ricky was the signal to start the night portion of the cross-Canada debauchery, which I had told myself I would have nothing to do with after being invited countless times during the day. But I guess I was a little slow on my exit-stage-right cue, and before I knew it I had slid down the bench, making way for all the others who were no doubt also invited.

I soon found myself in another television series. I should have been paid as a film extra for this trip. First there was the heavy splat of a plastic bag of rolling tobacco being thrown down onto the Formica tabletop. Then swarthy hands sporting dirty fingernails and silver rings adorned with skulls grabbed the chromed edges of the table and lowered a dark denim-and-leather-vested hulk beside me. The grunt he made as he sat was barely audible over the din in the lounge car from the others and the jangle of metallic chains around his neck. I caught a whiff of his basilisk breath before he leaned back and cast a cold eye upon me as he threw one side of his Samson-length black hair over a shoulder, exposing yet more hair on his rugged, acne-scarred face.

I made a meek obligatory offering of my menthols to the Klingon, which he met with a fortified French-Canadian accent that said, "Non." Oh, I wasn't about to use any of my cereal-box French with this guy, but when he gestured for me to roll my own out of his bag I greedily dug in. The Klingon's expression lit up when I rolled the first of what would turn out to be many with one hand; all those years of rolling foam ear plugs in the factory sure came in handy. I could have rolled one in each hand at the same time, but you have to understand that I didn't want to bring attention to myself. I should have known better with the Trailer Park Boys around.

Now if I was under any positive illusions about my weight, the crowd in that lounge put me in my place. When I got up to leave a cry of "Big Red!" burst out, and I had to walk a gauntlet of additional cheering, backslapping, high-fives, and hair messing. The moniker "Big Red" referred to my ever-present red jacket, and of course the belly underneath it. No, my adherence to the Document had not made me skinny.

By the time I got back to my coach seat, my attempt at a bit of stationary Sun Run training had doused my emotional well-being with cold water and had physically ruined me with all the cola and smoke and all.

Twenty-four hours later, Shelly was walking me through the massive sandstone archway of the Edwardian-classicist Vancouver train station and giving me the standard post-trip debriefing on whether my mother was dead or alive. Once we got to Shelly's vehicle I told her I had to go back in to use the washroom, which produced a look of annoyance. When I returned, she was sitting in the passenger seat waiting for me to drive, as is the custom when we are together since Shelly pretty much drives Greater Vancouver for a living, while my commuting is limited to the neighbourhood. I slid in behind the wheel and checked my pocket for my keys, then another pocket, then another. When I told Shelly I needed to go back to the train again to look for my keys, the disclosure was met with dead silence.

Getting back on the train was a hassle, but eventually I found someone in charge who let me board, and I was able to search all the nooks and crannies that I had encountered on my travels. I didn't find much, not even empty whisky bottles, since a cleaning crew had already done a first sweep of the car I had been in. I stood up after one final scrounge, placed a hand in my jacket pocket, and out came my keys. Oh, boy. The trip had left me as daft as a brush without bristles.

On my third trip under the archway, I saw Shelly scooting on her tiptoes out to the parking meter next to Thornton Park, plugging it, then scooting back to the driver's seat. I had wanted so much to yell out that I was there and all was right, but I thought better of it and instead slinked up to the passenger side of the vehicle and assumed my position. With the door safely closed, I told her I had found the keys in my pocket and reminded her that seeing her made my heart beat like thunder. Shelly rolled her big eyes then threw the car in gear and hit the throttle. My temple bounced off the headrest, leaving me woozy. I think I would have preferred a slap upside the head.

I couldn't get out of bed and into my running gear fast enough the next morning. This was it, the last day to register for the Sun Run, and I still didn't know if I could run. I mean, I knew I used to be able to run, but that was over a week earlier, so the question was, could I still run? By the time I got the heart pumping with the excitement of getting dressed, shooed the dog away while doing the stretching exercises, rearranged my underwear while running to the Sungod Track, and did a few Toller Cranston hand rolls, the run was over and I was standing at the back door feeling all dressed up with nowhere to go.

My plan had been to do one lap around the track—you know, to test myself—come home, then make an assessment. Well, even after going I didn't feel as if I had gone. Where was the sweat? The heavy breathing? I didn't even remember feeling any strain on Berm's Peak. The effortlessness of the test left me feeling like I was a runner, a bona fide runner, someone with bulletproof knees who didn't think each footfall would be his last. Yes, I could now hold my head high and go downtown to register knowing that I, Dave Hutchinson, while not yet a contender, was a somebody, someone who could run the Vancouver Sun Run. The door then opened a smidgen, and Shelly peered out and asked if I had lost my key.

Sun Run

The Vancouver Sun Run 2003
Kilometre 1
6 minutes 4 seconds

If I had woken up any faster on the morning of the Sun Run, my instant-on state could have been passed off as being a three-band transistor. My normal start-up process is more like a vacuum tube, with the synapses firing up with a warm hint of energy and taking a moment to attain an overall luminescence of life. Of course Shelly would disagree with this parallelism by pointing out that I contain far more gas than any vacuum tube. Nevertheless, I found myself dressed in my running outfit in record-shattering time, giving me more mirror time to scrutinize the accessories required for the day. More mirror time for me is never a good thing, but I felt it was imperative that I look the part on my Sun Run debut.

Looking the part meant wearing the white T-shirt issued at registration with the Tiko Kerr artistic rendering of a Sun Run start. It is a fabulous painting of fifty thousand participants, mostly represented by a kaleidoscope of round coloured dabs under billowing strings of balloons as they queue on Georgia Street. The scene, including the adjacent buildings, is depicted with the Tiko Kerr paradigm-bending wavy brush stroke. In fact it was this wave thing that was the hardest part of registering. The woman at the registration desk asked me what my expected finish time would be. Well, I wasn't prepared to give up such personal information, so I fired back a couple of my own questions. The woman replied that she didn't want to have a conversation with me, she just wanted to register me. I guess I was a touch obstinate, but I'm not belligerent, so I took my form off to the side of the hotel lobby under her watchful eye and thought the whole thing through.

Oh, sure, I had heard about the Sun Run wave start, but I figured it was done on a first-come basis. You know, two thousand runners at a time being allowed to start, then after a few minutes the next two thousand runners starting. The wave start being done according to a runner's ability never occurred to me, but as I stood pretending to shop at a rack of running clothes for sale, I had to decide which of my two times to give.

I had thought this whole timing thing through as well, but I never thought I would need to tell anybody beforehand. Over the years, on the day after every Sun Run, the most popular question I'd overheard from people who have just met each other at work, in the mall, or on the street was "What was your time?" It is a diabolical question, really, and should be banned from our cultural greeting exchange. You see, the answer requires a degree of precision and exactness that pretty much stifles then snuffs out any possibility of giving a creative answer. And why is that? Because the runners receive timing chips that they attach to their running shoes with plastic ties, and the *Vancouver Sun* publishes the finishing times of all participants in the paper after the run.

So, I wasn't looking forward to the moment when someone asks me a question he quite possibly knows the answer to. It's not that I'm a chronic liar or anything, it's just that the question removes the ability to give a generalized answer such as, "I ran a good race," or "It was a personal best, man," or "Even I gave up and walked the second half." The person asking the question isn't looking for evasiveness or excuses, he is looking for the time, and that's all he wants to hear. And you know—just as you know Greater Vancouver has a monsoon season—that he will have a seeded time of forty-five minutes or less.

I stared at the form, with its option of six different wave-start positions based on expected finish time. Should I go with my pro-rated Run for Life time of seventy minutes, or should I use a conservative estimation of eighty minutes? I was stymied; each of my estimates was in a different wave-start position. White or purple, follower or leader, full of it or great prognosticator, passee or passer? Oh, I winced at that last thought, then caught the registration lady looking at me again. Most likely she thought I didn't like the prices; hopefully she didn't think I was stealing and had just hurt myself on an errant pin in my pocket.

In reality I was dealing with the cold, hard truth of my physical and mental capabilities, and what fun was that? I ticked off the final runners category before the walkers and dragged my butt back to the registration table. "Eighty minutes," I said as I handed her the form. She shuffled around a few papers, then got my T-shirt, timing chip, and bib number, which she promptly turned over and, pointing to the wording on the back side, said with a certain amount of satisfaction, "It's called the pink section on your bib." My eyes downshifted to the bifocal portion of my glasses, and sure enough the fine print said, "Pink numbers line up on Howe Street." Oh, I guess I had that coming. It was pansy enough that I had to line up at the back, but it was an insult to injury that I had been identified with the pink crowd.

I don't have a mano a mano tattoo on my arm with some extended acronym for the hockey expression "Wanna go?" but I did have my bib, number 40652, pinned to my chest. For the record, it was purple in colour and identified as such on all other literature, including Tiko Kerr's painting, and it looked mighty fine in the mirror that morning. So did the contrasting long-sleeved red shirt that was under the T-shirt. I adjusted my white cap, then took the ensemble into the backyard to test it in the weather. It was dark out and threatening to rain, and it felt a bit cool on the bare legs, but after checking that my chip was attached and that the mesh-panelled babies were double tied, I decided that the long sleeves were a bit much. Back inside I went and switched to a short-sleeved shirt, red of course.

Moments later, still feeling as if I was overheating, I realized that the paper bib, which was sitting high on my chest, was making me hot and bothered. I reattached it lower towards the belly and stepped back outside. Now I felt a bit cold, so in I went again and took a long hard look at my running jacket. After sizing it up, I grabbed it and began folding it in on itself, then I strapped the small pouch around my waist. On my walk towards the back door for another weather check, I stopped and took the pouch off; the sensation of its bobbing around in the small of my back had been far too distracting, and I began to think about wearing the running jacket full time.

It was at this point that I felt like a pinball that had landed in a mid-board hole named inexperience, with flashing lights and all. I didn't know where, when, or how fast I would pop out of the hole with a clothing answer, so I decided to go with what previous experience had taught me. Although it seemed like the sort of day to execute this pouch trick, the problem was I had never practiced running with it on, and I had learned long ago not to introduce something this radical to my routine on any big day. Then on one last pinball bounce outside for a weather check, my mind said I felt a bit overheated once again. Whether this was the case or not I didn't know, but at the time the confirmation was oh so soothing.

It was time to do some light exercising and wake the gang, so I fired up the tubes and put on a CD of hockey arena anthems. Shelly was the first to saunter down the stairs to the thump of a Bachman-Turner Overdrive song, followed by Emma with her hair messed in every manner and dragging her bedspread behind her. Both gave me a sleepy-eyed cursory glance with no accompanying words as they continued on to the kitchen.

The third figure down the stairs did not give me the same deference and stopped in the middle of the stairs, took in the exercise routine for a moment, then stretched out herself as she gave me a long, half-yawning, "Give me a break." It was Nancy the powerbabe's daughter, who had slept over and would accompany Shelly, Emma, and I down to the Sun Run. Nancy was going to bus down with her Sun Run training group and meet up with us after the run to get a ride back to North Delta.

After breakfast, getting everybody out the door was easier than usual when I gave them the option of humming the Hockey Night in Canada theme song, singing "O Canada," or piling into the vehicle for the ride downtown. Yes, I realize that if at any future point in my life, should my family sit me down and point-blank tell me they can't take it anymore, I'll buy a new "let's move out" CD, probably volume II.

The Sunday morning ride downtown was easy, quiet, and uneventful as all my passengers fell asleep during the thirty-five-minute trip to B.C. Place Stadium. I became a bit concerned when I pulled into the parking lot and had a choice of any of the parking spaces. Each and every day I try my best to avoid situations like this, where I stand a chance of being really, really, super-colossally wrong. I did a quick look around for signs indicating that the lot was closed (for the groundbreaking of a new condo tower or something). With no evidence of impending dynamite explosions, I selected a nice corner space and hopped out of the vehicle.

I thought I was vibrating with anticipation but could have been shivering in the cold as I waited for the gang to pile out and give me a send-off. No sooner did the final door close than I did a herky-jerky two-step skip followed by a three-step walk towards the Sun Run start, which was more than a kilometre away. It was as if the perplexing parking situation had set my motor running and I was having trouble governing the throttle.

I continued with the strange gait until I caught up with a group of other Sun Run participants walking down Robson Street. It felt good to see these comrades in arms, who corroborated that all watches and clocks in my household were set correctly and that I hadn't misread the calendar.

I pulled away from the pack a block from my wave-start access point to do some more stretching. As I gently tweaked one muscle then another, I could not help but notice that the scene around me was looking a lot like the Stanley Cup riot of 1994. Actually, this crowd was better dressed, or at least the cost per outfit was higher, plus I didn't smell or see any joints being passed around, nor did I hear any of alcohol's accompanying tell-tale sounds of glass bottles tinkling on cement. On further reflection I didn't hear any profanity, yahoos, or stomach retching either.

Now before you think I was dodging rubber bullets and waving off pepper spray attacks as some front-line combatant, I should point out where Shelly and I lived back in 1994. It was a marvellous first-floor corner suite on a popular West End corner, with wall-to-wall double-hung windows. With the windows open to two different streets it was like having a front-row seat to the marshalling area, which included all the sights, sounds, and smells in stereo. In fact as Shelly and I sat watching game seven between the Canucks and the Rangers, we heard the refrain, "Going to the riot?" start during the second period. I am still shocked to this day at how the game's outcome was a moot point and that a confrontation had become inevitable.

What these two seemingly dissimilar crowds had in common was a constant stream of walkers from every direction converging on one location, coupled with a sense of menace. Menace of varying degrees mind you, but let me tell you I could feel the malice clogging my craw. This wasn't a fireworks crowd, a football crowd, or even a car-racing crowd that congregates for the sole purpose of being entertained. The 1994 riot crowd and the 2003 Sun Run crowd *were* the entertainment, and both marched towards their destinations with a performance-driven intensity worthy of settling the deed. At least that was my working theory at the time to explain why the shakes had returned and why the loops of my laces were doing their best imitation of a jitterbug. Of course after having put so much thought and effort into my running wear that morning, I was loath to admit that the cold weather had anything to do with it.

It felt good to be walking again as I made my way along the final block before joining up with the purple-bibbed crowd. I rounded the corner of Robson and Howe to an unsettling scene that required my immediate consideration. At the end of the block on Georgia Street was, live and in person, the expected mass assemblage of humanity. When I realized I would not be able to join them on Georgia Street because the lineup continued on past Howe Street, forcing me to line up perpendicular to it, next to the Art Gallery, I did a quick Toller Cranston hand roll. I took this escape from having to negotiate with my sardine-can neurosis as a positive sign, but it was the commotion in the middle of the block that was unsettling. There was a long row of portable toilets, each with an accompanying long line of fellow runners. Should I go, or should I go? The deliberation was short because once I took a few steps towards my wave-start position, I found myself drawn past the portables and glomming onto the rest of the assembled mass, much like the gravitational forces apparent in a lava lamp.

From this vantage point I was able to look out over the crowd before me, capture the melody of an unseen live band, and listen to snippets of conversation from three sides. It was minutes before the 9:00 a.m. start, maybe forty minutes before the purple wave would go, and I was so pleased with myself for taking extra time out for stretching before getting to this point. And then the staring started.

No one stares at me. I mean, putting the De Niro tough guy stuff aside, no one stares at me. I don't even stare at me. So there I was with two girls and a guy in front of me, taking turns staring. Oh, goodness, this made me tense, and soon my hands roamed my body looking for anomalies.

I was in the middle of a slow 100 percent hand coverage of my body, as practiced in my youth swishing mosquitoes away, when the entire crowd erupted into a chorus of cheers. Thinking that my start calculations were off, I prepared to run, but there was no shoulder dipping, no elbows arching, and no forward motion by my body or anybody. Instead, the only movement was thousands of heads that had swivelled in an upward motion.

I followed the direction they were looking, up to a large window near the top of a high-rise hotel. There, standing in profile with an arched back in a dramatic pose, was a tall young man with wavy blonde hair—you know, Duran Duran style—standing buck naked. I dare say he had a runner's body, his winter-white skin taut against its angular frame. The crowd upped the cheering when he pirouetted in the window, giving us a full frontal view before he sashayed his way to an exit stage right.

Now *that* changed the atmosphere amongst the masses, even if we all had to endure a pesky drizzle on our faces as we scanned the upper floors of the hotel for an encore. Holy stage presence, let there be no doubt about it. We got more, but it wasn't really an encore, it was more like act two. The crowd roared again in approval at the nudity, but this time it was from a lower-floor window by a different young man, who had a bronzed, hairless, muscular body and close-cropped black hair. This lower-floor flasher lacked the refined, fluid movement of act one, as his inchoate display included jumping jacks of all things.

It was at this point that I started looking around for any sign of us all being put on, and it was only then that I saw why I was being stared at earlier. The people weren't looking at me, they were looking at the massive crowd that had formed behind me. But before I could let my own fears take hold, I got distracted as the crowd went wild when the first flasher returned, this time with a prop. The lanky blonde with a Godiva slink in his step gave us the profile look once more, but this time he was talking coyly on the black hotel phone. The blonde made the most of his captive audience by giving a sultry performance, which included entrancing us all with the whipping movements of his long coiled cord.

When the third act was over, I fully expected a helicopter to manoeuvre its way through the concrete canyon of Georgia Street, trailing a banner for some diva show at a local gay bar. It didn't happen, not because it couldn't happen but more likely because it was an oversight since this really was a case of the truth being stranger than fiction. Instead, all we got coming out of the sky was more rain.

Moments later the truth was so strange it felt phony. My group had been marshalled out onto Georgia Street, and I was standing in the middle of the street looking into the HSBC building at its public art of a pendulum suspended from the ceiling over a stationary pedestal. While this all felt a touch surreal, the phony part was the amount of space I had around me. I had plenty of room to snap a telephone cord or at the very least swing a jockstrap, and this didn't feel right since I had tossed and turned all night preparing for the exact opposite. In the midst of this personal space check, the purple-bibbed crowd began to surge forward, and I had to do a quick two-step just to retain the new-found space and of course stay with the pack.

The surge forward turned into a slow trot, but out of the corner of my eye I saw a few people dart sideways while they pulled a layer of clothing up over their heads. The clothing was then thrown to the top of a temporary chain-link fence on the outer edge of the course. As the runners returned to the main body of the crowd, they pounded their fists in the air to the music emanating from the P.A. system of a live band we were about to pass. I noticed many other pieces of outerwear pushed through the openings of the fence, then I checked the other side of the street and saw that fence in the same condition.

I was pondering the fact that all the apparel was some shade of castaway grey when I heard what sounded like a live downed power line. I would never have stepped over, on, or even under the source of electronic noise coming from the Sun Run start line if hundreds of other people weren't doing so before my eyes. Still, when it came time for me to cross and activate the electronic chip on my shoe, I could not help but shorten my stride and clench my gluteus maximus (and of course the medius and minimus, too) as I squeezed my inner thighs together.

When I brought my head up after opening a small plastic bag that contained toothpaste and placing a dab on my tongue—a carry-over from having to brush my teeth before each training run—and pushing the lap-counter function on my watch, what I saw was exhilarating. The walkers had taken to the right side of the street, while the fast runners took to the left, leaving me to absorb what was remaining into my personal space, an ocean of concrete that appeared to be mine straight through to the horizon, where it emptied into Lost Lagoon. Oh, the mesh-panelled babies needed no coaxing. It was go time, and I did my best Ben Johnson imitation as I shot up the gap.

After I had re-adjusted myself below the belt, taken in some architectural landscaping, and caught a glimpse of a single-engine Otter seaplane landing in Coal Harbour, I could feel my fellow purple bibbers, who were mostly walkers at this point, drifting to the left. This ended my sightseeing tour and brought my attention back to the course, where I saw a big 1 KM sign. I then retrieved from my watch the first split time and ended up eyeballing the results since I couldn't believe what I was seeing: six minutes and four seconds. I had barely run a seven-minute kilometre in training, so how did I do a six-minute one now? Then again, what in the world was I doing running almost a five-minute kilometre?

The Vancouver Sun Run 2003
Kilometre 2
6 minutes 10 seconds

I started off the second kilometre dazed and confused as I tried to figure out where I went wrong with the speed thing and only snapped out of it when someone shook a cowbell in my face and someone else demanded a high-five. Fans, my first who did not require sleepy-time kisses. This part of the course was like entering a raucous, twisty bendy funnel as it made its way from the hard angular surfaces of Georgia Street to the soft natural coverings in the outer rim of Stanley Park. I adjusted my line of running towards the middle of the course to reduce the chance of further fan contact, then I continued with the assessment of my speed. Now, there were lots of reasons I was concerned about having a great first split time, with the first being speed kills, doesn't it? Oh, sure, to say nothing about my inability to foresee such circumstances, what about the circumstances themselves? For goodness' sake, my body wasn't prepared for six-minute kilometres, and when the second kilometre time confirmed a trend, there was no doubt in my mind that I stood a chance of not making it out of this race alive.

The Vancouver Sun Run 2003
Kilometre 3
16 minutes 13 seconds

It was at this point that I felt psychologically defeated. My inexperience with running in large crowds had reduced all my training and preparation to mere sidebars, as it was apparent I was running on primal instinct alone. So while I was still shaking my head at the second split time, I pulled up and gathered my thoughts while I stood in a lineup to use a portable toilet.

It crossed my mind that my speed was based on the fact that I was just running to go to the bathroom, but I thought better of it after factoring in the whole Ben Johnson start-line action of bolting at the buzz. I moved up a position at the creak and slam of a plastic door while I continued to figure out what had gone wrong. What was with this whole Ben Johnson fixation at this point of my training initiative, anyway? I figured it had to be some sort of Poh-Poh–like sign that needed yet another sign before an interpretation could be made. So while I was on the lookout (you know, for something like a women's track suit hanging up in the portable toilet), the door slamming went on and on.

You see, when Pete McMartin was covering the Seoul Olympics in 1988, he reported that Ben Johnson had worn a women's track suit when he emerged from the area where he had provided a urine sample. So I had pretty much resigned myself to quitting should there be a women's size large track suit hanging on the back of the door, when with the suddenness of a master of ceremonies' appearance at a three-ring circus, the door was flung open, stressing its hinges to the max. Out strutted a man of pomp wearing grimy jeans with holes in them, scuffed brown work boots, two plaid shirts, one of each colour and an unzipped hooded grey nylon parka. He then laughed the big laugh at all those ogling him.

I was next, but before I took a step forward I stared in amazement at the man, who then joined an equally scruffy woman who had been waiting for him. Together they enjoyed one more roaring laugh before they headed away from the course and into the park. A line from Timothy Taylor's novel *Stanley Park* extended my immobilization while I reviewed it: "Then lagoon traffic changed direction like a freak tide." One of the characters in Taylor's story had spent time observing the homeless in Stanley Park. I'd always admired the simile but never thought I would live it to the extent that it had an impact on my bladder.

Well, after hearing a few "hurry ups" I took my turn. Once inside the portable I looked around, then up then down, but there wasn't a track suit to be found. Of course, my final thought before I exited was that the homeless guy took it.

I started off this third kilometre by not having a drink at the water station. I was trying to get myself back on my game plan, which in this case meant drinking only at the midway point, which I figured would approximate my real-life training conditions. The cedar, fir, and hemlock trees in the park shielded us from the rain through this portion of the run. Yes, us. Somehow I had ended up in the middle of a pack of runners, who were blazing along in the left lane of all things. I tried to see whom we were passing since there were also some runners over on the right, but I found it far too treacherous to get a good look since the pack really was packed and my full concentration was needed if only to stay upright. Plus we were moving so fast that way over there on the right was nothing but a blur.

I did dare to look at the immediate runners to my sides in the pack and saw nothing but hard bodies. None of them were over thirty years of age. Alarm bells started going off, and I began to question why I had bothered to stop and gather myself if I wasn't going to follow through on the contingency plan of finding someone in my age group to tag along with. I didn't know what to do. Should I slow down and be normal or continue to kick butt on the flattest, prettiest stretch of road I'd ever run on?

As if I didn't have enough factors to contend with as I contemplated the wisdom of my running tactics, I now had to include the excitement factor. When we came out of the park, this represented not only the end of kilometre three but also the entrance to my old stomping grounds at English Bay. The heartwarming sight of long lines of immaculately placed logs on the groomed beach while the bay lapped its soft, smooth edges expunged any stinking conservative notions I had of taking it easy. This was it, the pinnacle of my slavish devotion to the Document. Hey, I was in the left lane, I was on home turf—it was show time. Moments later I had to hold myself back from throwing my arms in the air, facing the treetops, and declaring the extent of my glory. Oh, I was tearing that course up.

The Vancouver Sun Run 2003
Kilometre 4
6 minutes 24 seconds

On the morning of April 13, 2003, had you been a hungover, binged-out Polish sailor leaning on the rail of a rusted freighter anchored in English Bay, you would have seen an older African-Canadian male make his move on me in front of the English Bay bathhouse.

I felt his presence on my left side while I looked beyond that rusted freighter at the view looming on the horizon, from Wreck Beach to Point Atkinson, of a castaway grey curtain of rain that was headed for the city. I attempted to fend him off with a Landy left shoulder check, but to no avail. He repelled my formidable stare with a Roger Neilson–inspired wave of white-towel power as he wiped his perspiration-soaked bald head.

He was an extra, extra large man whose lumbering stride made me look as if I were back to tiptoeing on the Sungod Track again. Oh, and that towel. He was using it relentlessly on me as he brought it up with a wave every thirty seconds or so to wipe his newel-post-like head. There was no doubt in my mind that a challenge had been thrown down, and I felt confident that the good doctor and his Document had brought me to this point fully prepared for what needed to be done next. You know, feel free to up the ante, the thought of injury shouldn't hold you back—at least that was my interpretation of the signs.

The good doctor would be Dr. Doug Clement, the former Canadian Olympic runner who had developed the original running program that the 2003 training Document was based on. Of course, the sport medicine physician's graduated program was great and all, but my confidence at that moment for taking on what needed to be done stemmed from the doctor's wife, Diane. With the appearance of "the Towel of Nam," as I would come to call the man with the shaved

270

head later in the run, I could now reinterpret the whole Ben Johnson thing from the first kilometres of the Sun Run.

"The Towel of Nam" represented Ben Johnson, of course, but it was my rethinking of my fixation on the women's track suit that soothed any deep-seated fears I may have had about picking up the challenge. You see, the track suit had belonged to Diane Clement, team manager of the 1988 Canadian Olympic track team. Diane, who was a sprinter on the 1956 Canadian Olympic team, lent Ben her track suit when they discovered that Ben's official Canadian Olympic track suit had been left behind in Canada and he had to make a media appearance. Once I considered that Diane was a founding member of the 1985 Vancouver Sun Run, all the signs seemed to point in the right direction. There was no need for a Poh-Poh second opinion. My fate was sealed and I was good to go.

When we came to the bandstand in Alexander Park, I made a subtle course change and veered towards the bay. "The Towel of Nam" stayed on my shoulder, confirming my suspicion that the challenge was on, thus eliminating the need for a verification loop around the inukshuk. I kept a wary eye on the challenger as we headed east on Beach Avenue. He had tremendous pace and rhythm, so much so that I felt on the verge of being hypnotized by the massive piston-like strokes of his strides and the flywheel precision of the towel that went way up, did a quick twirl, then came way down. I planned to push forward the challenge and curtail all this towel waving where Beach Avenue split off to the right, with the straight portion becoming Pacific Boulevard.

In the old days, if I phoned Dad after dinner and he wasn't home, I would walk down the block and usually meet up with him on a park bench on this corner. Back then there was no sign of the palm trees that I had set my sights on during this Sun Run. When we came upon the exotic foliage, I took advantage of the small incline that Beach Avenue incurred and put some space between us. Oh, my breathing got a little out of control with the excitement at being so smart, so physically capable, and so forthright in my intentions. It didn't last long, though, and by the time I closed to within site of the Stealth fighter jet rooflines of the Vancouver Aquatic Centre, signalling the end of the fourth kilometre, I could feel the wind turbulence of that towel once more on my left side.

The Vancouver Sun Run 2003
Kilometre 5
7 minutes 8 seconds

With "the Towel of Nam" back on my shoulder, I threw him a simple yet vicious Landy left shoulder check. He seemed impervious to it, but I had to make some attempt at letting him know there would be another push coming.

The original pack that had formed up in Stanley Park were nowhere to be seen. I had no idea if they were behind us cooling their heels in a portable toilet lineup or ahead of us in the warm confines of B.C. Place Stadium at the finish line. It was a bit chaotic out there on the course, with some people walking slower than you, some running faster, and—the worst—people transitioning from running to walking right in front of you. So it was tough keeping tabs on everybody when you had to keep your wits about you. Plus I was busy getting myself mentally prepared for any counter-push and of course getting set for my own next push, where Beach Avenue became a dead end.

The course width had become a bit constricted, with walkers forcing us onto the left sidewalk as we kept our pace strong and steady. We were now within jostling distance of one another, and in fact, at times I could feel the towel touch me in its never-ending quest to keep the newel post dry. I was tempted to ask if he would like to say hello to my little friend, then finger-flick him upside the head, but I didn't. Instead, I used the irritation of a towel flick here and a towel flick there for additional inspiration as I prepared to unleash the strength of my running repertoire against him.

I had no plans of making this a photo finish. I was going to demoralize him at the five-kilometre mark with my hill-climbing ability. Yes, I am from North Delta, and as a matter of course I trained on hills, none of this namby-pamby by-the-sea flat stuff. When I saw how the shadow of the Granville Street Bridge had darkened Beach Avenue's dead end, it was my belief that this little charade of running together would soon be over.

I forced the two of us to close in tight on a band that was playing under the bridge as I made a hard left turn, then found myself more than pleased with what I saw and, even more important, after a few steps what I felt.

Oh, I had driven this short, steep section many times and parked there on a few occasions while having dinner in the neighbourhood. I'd even been there to pick up my impounded car, but I had never walked it in its entirety. The steep grade forced an abrupt posture change that had more in common with skiing downhill than running uphill, and I let the thigh muscles take over.

Within ten feet I was running solo; it was as if the big man had run into a concrete support piling. The immediate success of my plan invigorated me, and I powered my way up to Pacific Boulevard in an effortless fashion. Once I was out from under the cover of the bridge and cruising through a flat portion of the course before the next grade on Burrard Bridge, I couldn't help but smile as I brought my arm up to mark the five-kilometre split time. It was mission accomplished.

The Vancouver Sun Run 2003
Kilometre 6
8 minutes 1 second

I might as well have been sitting in an armchair at the corner of Burrard and Pacific Boulevard, having a coffee while imparting to my boxing friend Lenny for the hundredth time in my most contemptuous and annoying manner why I call him "Shake and Bake," when "the

Towel of Nam" blew by. Oh, sweet Patsy Cline, I'll never forget the shock of seeing the back of his broad shoulders for the first time, framed against the pastel archway of the Burrard Bridge. I then calculated the distance and degree of incline to that archway before I drew a bead on the towel flailing at his side and changed my foot landing forward to the ball of my toes. It was go time.

I must admit the grade of the bridge didn't intimidate me. I had seen the same grade before (and the one kilometre or so distance) on 112th Street from 72nd Avenue to the Sungod Recreation Centre. I knew I was capable, I felt good, and I was more than ready to respond to the challenge. What did intimidate me, though, was the speed with which I was passed and even more so the gap that it produced between us.

When I passed him there were no Landy left shoulder checks. No singing, "Na, na, na, na hey, hey, hey." No Toller Cranston hand rolls. No nothing. I just kept going straight through to the apex of the grade, then kept on going on the downside. With the cruise control set to high, I looked out over English Bay and saw that the curtain of rain was almost upon this section of the course. It looked bad, but I didn't need this as an incentive to keep the throttle down—not wanting to see that white towel again took care of that.

I was looking forward to a good six-kilometre split time when I noticed in the distance a young Oriental woman break away from her husband, who was pushing a baby carriage, and join the conductor of a brass band on his podium. She finished the song with some vigorous arm waving before jumping off and skipping back to her family. I was taking delight in her jolly good cheer when a cramp wrenched my left side with a pain that had me bending over and in a full stagger. As lightning fast as the cramp came on, the end of my challenge with "the Towel of Nam" was far faster as survival mode kicked in.

The Vancouver Sun Run 2003
Kilometre 7
9 minutes 2 seconds

It was at this point—when I was in agony—that I could fully appreciate thirteen straight weeks of training. My legs kept moving (they did not know any better), but my mind became clouded and I remember not being able to hear properly. Somehow I was able to concentrate and implement a few techniques I had read about in the paper, which I had used successfully in the past on minor cramps. I changed my pace, as if I had any choice, then began to exhale every time my left foot planted. I would do this until the cramp went away. The pain had become tolerable, but only because a soothing flat section had awaited me when I turned left onto 2nd Avenue. It was when the course turned up Fir Street and its touch of grade that I began to look for a piece of lawn to lie down and give up on, the wetter the better. I was oh so close to being tapped out, but then the competition pulled up alongside and pushed the Cuyler Goodwill end point out a bit further.

"Hey, man, you all right?" asked the guy with the towel.

I looked up at him, over my left shoulder of course, then squeaked out a feeble sounding, "Why?"

"You were jibberin' something fierce, man."

I had to ask, knowing I would never see the guy again in my life and that I was beyond embarrassment, "Was it Chinese?" Of course, I didn't know Mandarin or Cantonese, never did.

"Oh, no. I served in Nam. It sounded more Vietnamese. Hey, man, drink that water up and take care of yourself."

I looked back at my right hand, which was sticking straight out in the far forward position, and in it was the cup of water I had received from an elderly Oriental woman wearing a blue quilted jacket. I gingerly brought it to my lips and took a single sip, then continued running with it as if the second half of the Sun Run was some sort of waiters' race. "The Towel of Nam" moved on ahead of me. He wasn't going all that fast; it was more a case of my trudge being slower than his.

When the course took a left turn at 4th Avenue, I took the opportunity to look back down Fir Street to see if an elderly Oriental woman wearing a blue quilted jacket was still handing out water. It had to be Poh-Poh. Who else but a fictional character could have brought a Denny Boyd simile to life? "She gave me her hand. It was like holding a small silk bag of marbles." This was the sensation I had when our hands cupped for the passing of the gift of water.

Obviously my overexertion protection had failed me. I took another sip and looked over at the seven-foot-high stone numerals that were erected in the park beside Granville Bridge to celebrate the city's one hundredth anniversary. Even with the ominous scenario of the interior edges of the mesh-panelled babies clipping each other, I was still able to retain a strong suspicion that I had been operating in a realm beyond my comprehension.

I remember thinking, *What's next, a hallucination of Suzette Meyers sitting on the numeral one?* Oh, she would be in a contemplative thinker's posture, slowly rocking one leg over the other while wearing knee-high chocolate brown equestrian boots. On the first zero, Denny Boyd would be standing upright, black boots and all (including shiny metal toe taps), with his chin to the clouds in his best "Sky Pilot" pose, while his Eric Burdon bangs did a soft curl just past his right eyebrow. Oh, sure, and Pete McMartin would be naked and lying vertical on the second zero, his runners covering his private parts as in some Burt Reynolds retro-style photo shoot.

I tossed the cup to the ground when I visualized McMartin giving me a smirk that mocked me to my soles. I punched the timer on my wrist, signalling the end of kilometre seven but more important the start of kilometre eight and a new beginning.

The Vancouver Sun Run 2003
Kilometre 8
6 minutes 9 seconds

I wish I could say that the probable course record for longest distance of a dropped cup from a water table on Fir Street to its landing under the Granville Bridge and the purging of all thoughts of McMartin's nakedness brought about an Elysium moment, but I can't. Instead, after piquing my subconscious with my representation of the Eric Burdon and The Animals song "Sky Pilot," I was now battling the song's sound of bagpipes and its terrifying Hollywood-enhanced whine of an aircraft in an uncontrolled nosedive.

Despite this, I was feeling better because the cramp had gone, and it was here at the beginning of kilometre eight that I held another frank conference call with myself to myself about myself. At the call's conclusion, I knew what I had to do. It had come down to this: if I was going to finish this whole running initiative with more swagger than stagger then I would need to–as Shelly was fond of pointing out– "...face the music and dance."

I searched for a different tune. I wanted something uplifting, something with rhythm, something to smooth out any trouble that may lie ahead. A few soothing Toller Cranston hand rolls later, the horrific "Sky Pilot" sound effects stopped when I cued another sixties sound from the jukebox of my mind with the Petula Clark–like vocal harmonies of one-time British Columbia resident Nelly Furtado. I could hear Emma's tiny voice providing backup to the song "I'm Like a Bird" as it drifted through the hallways and down the stairs of our house. I latched on to it and immediately felt my feet lift a little higher off the pavement of 6th Avenue as I transitioned from mucking in the rain puddles to scudding along the tops of them.

Shelly always has a good laugh whenever I tell her about having another of my flying dreams. My last flying dream had me swooping the treetops of our backyard, which elicited this response from my wife: "Dave, you've got to stop hassling the crows and start soaring with the eagles." To me these are words of envy. You see, in this world not everybody dreams of flying. Shelly doesn't, but I bet Nelly Furtado does. For inquiring minds, my liftoff is done with the ankles; most flyers I know use their knees.

The course was all six lanes of 6th Avenue and all flat, providing ideal conditions for bringing home whatever you've got. This section of the course did have its peculiarities, though. Whereas for most of the course the walkers had stayed on the right-hand side, for this final section the left side became the preferred side to walk on. So I marked my second comeback of the race by chewing up the flat—oh, the glorious flat—on the Fairview Slope side of the street.

The Vancouver Sun Run 2003
Kilometre 9
6 minutes 17 seconds

At the beginning of the penultimate kilometre of the race, I saw some of the first runners returning from the finish line as they ran towards me. I was adjusting my line of running in order to let them pass when they suddenly veered left. When I caught up to them I could see that they had taken the 22 percent grade of Oak Street to exit the course, which triggered my gag reflex until it was positively out of sight. They don't build them like that anymore, thank goodness.

No sooner had I gotten my breathing back under control when the much-anticipated curtain of rain started to fall. It was a hard-driving, personal rain in that each and every drop demanded its presence be known to you on an individual basis with a heartfelt slap. I'd like to say that I buckled down and picked up the pace in order to outrun the rain, but that just wasn't an option: I was already flying along the straightest, flattest road that Vancouver has to offer at maximum speed. Oh, the mesh-panelled babies had never before had such an opportunity to showcase the speed aspect of their design, and they were making the most of it. Of course, they were getting outstanding support from my non-prescription-based inner cheerleading.

So while the convergence of shoe design and running performance was reaching a quantitative peak, the city's skyline had become indistinct. You would not have known that Greater Vancouver had any tall buildings let alone was nestled against the foot of the Coast Mountain range. The temperature may have been falling as well, but I had no way of knowing. I wasn't cold, but I could not feel my fingers touching my bare skin, a peculiar state I had been in since the Burrard Bridge. If I hadn't known better, I would have thought it to be a typical January winter's day.

There are many reasons why the Centennial Rocket near the Cambie Street Bridge captures my imagination, such as the unrestrained display of craftsmanship. The manufacturing process of a unique individual product is another. The time capsule in its base—have you ever seen or heard of one being opened?—is also interesting. The reason, though, that the twelve-foot-long art deco stylized rocket ship intrigues me the most is whether or not it should be there. It is a 1985 replica of the original built in 1936, and I'm thinking that maybe it should have been treated like a totem pole, with its limited lifespan an accepted fact. Of course, this line of thought has a few branches to it, which makes this piece of public art all the more compelling.

On this day, though, the rocket ship captured my imagination by boldly pointing the way to the final leg and the finish line over the Cambie Street Bridge. I throttled back at the base of the ship in order to save myself for a big push at the finish line, but when I started getting passed by everybody on the entrance ramp to the bridge, I had second thoughts and tried to readjust my speed. By the time the nine-kilometre mark appeared, this tactic was nothing more than a chimerical indulgence, and I had placed myself in a no-go situation. I couldn't deliver the final charge.

The Vancouver Sun Run 2003
Kilometre 10
8 minutes 3 seconds

I entered the tenth and final kilometre of the Vancouver Sun Run wishing for a can of oil. My knee caps were grinding bone on bone, and I was certain that a little intravenous oil drip was all that was needed to get me to the finish line looking like a runner. Oh, sure, I wanted to run across the finish line, but even with the downward slope of the bridge helping me along I knew I had to give it my all just to make it a close call.

When I heard the finish line buzz my fear grew, not for my private parts but that I might stride to the matted area covering the source of the electronic noise and collapse right smack on top of it, then curl up into a fetal position, causing all sorts of cellular carnage. My final words during the approach to the finish line were in the Ben Johnson vein: "Overshoot, overshoot."

I crossed the finish line, and my arms fell to my sides as I walked in an automaton daze towards a chip-removal queue. For goodness' sake, lie down, forget it—the legs wanted nothing to do with that. Once the electronic chip was snipped from my shoe by a Sun Run volunteer, I continued on towards B.C. Place Stadium. I didn't look around at the finish line well-wishers for my family. I didn't have to; the last time I saw them they hadn't been dressed to withstand a monsoon.

Round and round my legs carried my insensate torso down a ramp to the field level of the stadium. After taking in the height of the roof and how from this perspective it looked like the soiled underside of a mushroom in bondage, I tried to grab the nearest refreshment at hand, a yogurt cup off of a sample table. A man with a pleasant smile rebuffed my grab and insisted that I take a frozen yogurt that he had on his tray. Now I had never had yogurt before in my life, but I was willing to confess to anything, even to the pocketing of the Svend diamond, in order to have either the one on the table or the one on his tray.

I got my legs to stop walking, and I dug in with the wooden spoon. I didn't even blink when the spoon snapped. Instead, I held it high in the air and longed for anything moist to be clinging to its splintered edge. There wasn't, but as I held it up I noticed a commotion in the background, and when I brought my hand down I saw an older man tumbling down the final few steps on a stairway in the stands.

My stunned-state response was to squeeze my yogurt, which had the unintended effect of warming it up, and watch a crowd form as he was attended to. If the fallen runner's state of health could be determined by attributing a worsening severity value to each person who responded, then the sprawled figure in black tights was dead. My mind slipped to neutral and I could have stared at the morbidity of it all for the rest of the afternoon, but eventually the legs could not stay in one place any longer, and I moved out in search of the letter H in the stands. This was where my family would be.

I heard Shelly call out just as the partial spoon sectioned off a frozen chunk of yogurt, which was then shovelled into my mouth, "Hey, Rocketman, get over here." With the yogurt in my mouth and my wife's presence before me, I was overcome by a state of bliss like none other. I probably appeared mesmerized, maybe even dumbfounded, as I stood in silence staring at the cheerleaders in the front row, which included Nancy, the powerbabe. After the initial cheering they started to make their way down to field level as the powerbabe's daughter shouted out my card-playing name: "Hey, Dave Dirt, my mom kicked your butt."

I raised my yogurt cup in a symbolic cheer, then wondered how my time of seventy-nine minutes and thirty-one seconds would hold up against the masses. I would get my answer the next day when the *Vancouver Sun* published all the participants' results. In the meantime I took another stab at the yogurt as I walked back to the parking lot and reviewed the race. It would have been nice if I had known "the Towel of Nam's" name so I could check his time. It would have been nice if I had planned my bathroom breaks better. It would have been nice if I had allowed myself more water. It would have been nice if I had dressed properly.

All in all I had a lot of inexperience issues, but I was eternally grateful to be in the position at that moment of letting a happy ending ease its way into my very being. The fact that it had been much more challenging than anything I could have ever imagined made it that much better.

I had little energy to convey any of this at that moment, and what little I had was used to convince everybody to take an alternate route out of the stadium. I guess while the gang was waiting for me they had been planning a quick exit, which included taking the stairs. Well, of course I told them I had just seen a sign on the stairs. No, I didn't mention that it was a sign from Poh-Poh that said the way to the parking lot was via the ramp.

The End

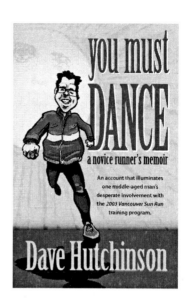

Author's biography

Dave Hutchinson, born in 1958 grew up in the Wolseley area of Winnipeg, Manitoba. It was the fierce prairie winds during those years that shaped the hairstyle that he wears today.

His Grandfather moved from Winnipeg to Vancouver in the 1950's and Dave followed his snow crusted footsteps thirty years later. His current residence is south of the Fraser River in the municipality of Delta. This is an officious designation though and Dave prefers to say that he is from North Delta.

ISBN 142514034-3

9 781425 140342